Psychiatry at a Glance

Psychiatry at a Glance

CORNELIUS KATONA

MD FRCPsych
Professor

MARY ROBERTSON

MD FRCPsych
Professor

Both of the Department of Psychiatry,
Royal Free and University College Medical School

SECOND EDITION

**Blackwell
Science**

© 1995, 2000 by
Blackwell Science Ltd
Editorial Offices:
Osney Mead, Oxford OX2 0EL
25 John Street, London WC1N 2BL
23 Ainslie Place, Edinburgh EH3 6AJ
350 Main Street, Malden
  MA 02148 5018, USA
54 University Street, Carlton
  Victoria 3053, Australia
10, rue Casimir Delavigne
  75006 Paris, France

Other Editorial Offices:
Blackwell Wissenschafts-Verlag GmbH
Kurfürstendamm 57
10707 Berlin, Germany

Blackwell Science KK
MG Kodenmacho Building
7–10 Kodenmacho Nihombashi
Chuo-ku, Tokyo 104, Japan

First published 1995
Second edition 2000
Reprinted 2000

Set by Graphicraft Ltd, Hong Kong
Printed and bound in Great Britain
at the Alden Press, Oxford and Northampton

The Blackwell Science logo is a
trade mark of Blackwell Science Ltd,
registered at the United Kingdom
Trade Marks Registry

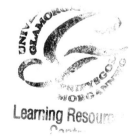
DISTRIBUTORS

Marston Book Services Ltd
PO Box 269
Abingdon, Oxon OX14 4YN
(*Orders*: Tel: 01235 465500
          Fax: 01235 465555)

USA
Blackwell Science, Inc.
Commerce Place
350 Main Street
Malden, MA 02148 5018
(*Orders*: Tel: 800 759 6102
              781 388 8250
          Fax: 781 388 8255)

Canada
Login Brothers Book Company
324 Saulteaux Crescent
Winnipeg, Manitoba R3J 3T2
(*Orders*: Tel: 204 837-2987)

Australia
Blackwell Science Pty Ltd
54 University Street
Carlton, Victoria 3053
(*Orders*: Tel: 3 9347 0300
          Fax: 3 9347 5001)

A catalogue record for this title
is available from the British Library

ISBN 0-632-05554-5

Library of Congress
Cataloging-in-publication Data

Katona, C. L. E. (Cornelius L. E.), 1954–
Psychiatry at a glance / Cornelius Katona,
Mary Robertson.—2nd ed.
    p.   ; cm.
Includes index.
ISBN 0–632–05554–5
1. Psychiatry.
I. Robertson, Mary M.
II. Title.
[DNLM: 1. Mental Disorders. 2. Psychiatry.
WM 140 K19p 1999]
RC454.K366   1999
616.89—dc21   99–044556

For further information on
Blackwell Science, visit our website:
www.blackwell-science.com

Contents

Introduction to the second edition

We are gratified by the very positive response we have received for *Psychiatry at a Glance* since its original publication in 1995. We are delighted that it received a commendation in the 1996 British Medical Association book awards. We are also pleased to note the publication of Japanese and Hungarian editions. *Psychiatry at a Glance* remains targeted primarily at the medical students who will be tomorrow's doctors. We very much hope that it will continue to meet their need for core psychiatric knowledge within their new curricula. The feedback we have received suggests that *Psychiatry at a Glance* is equally useful to nurses, social workers and psychologists and for psychiatric trainees. We have tried to consider the needs of all these groups of readers in preparing the second edition.

In the new edition we have taken the opportunity to correct any errors that have been brought to our notice by users of the book. We have also thoroughly revised the manuscript, both updating and reorganizing the text and figures. In so doing we have relied heavily on the goodwill of many expert colleagues, and take this opportunity of thanking Professor Michael King, Drs Abou-Saleh, Alcorn, Bruno, Channon, Cookson, Dein, Eapen, Freeman, Hassiotis, Hossain, Livingston, Morris, Norton, Orrell, Sensky, Shergill, Sturgeon, Turner, Tylee, Walker and Mr Geoffrey Smith for giving up their time, and for their helpful and constructive criticism. Responsibility for any errors and inaccuracies remains, of course, entirely ours. We have also written a new chapter on Risk Assessment and Management. In response to popular request we have added a 'further reading' list and multiple choice questions.

As before we would like to thank Philippa Katona and John Ludgate for their continued patience, support and helpful comments.

Cornelius Katona
Mary Robertson
London, October 1999

Introduction to the first edition

We have written *Psychiatry at a Glance* at the instigation of many of our students, with the intention of providing a text that is concise, easily portable and enjoyable to read. The book summarizes the content of a comprehensive lecture course in psychiatry. It is targeted primarily at clinical undergraduate medical students doing their psychiatry attachment and revising for final MB examinations. It should also be useful for psychiatric trainees revising for their MRCPsych Part 1 (or equivalent first specialist examination).

We have both been MB final (and MRCPsych Part 1) examiners for several years, as well as being involved in the design and delivery of the UCL Medical School undergraduate and postgraduate psychiatry courses. We are confident of having provided all the information content relevant to the psychiatry element of the GMC 'core' undergraduate medical curriculum. The diagrams encapsulate all a medical student needs to know in order to pass—and should also help in last minute revision! The text supplements this sufficiently to provide enough for a student to do well.

We are also aware that, as psychiatric care moves into the community, a basic knowledge of psychiatry is increasingly important for a variety of clinical practitioners. *Psychiatry at a Glance* should provide a useful introduction to the specialty for psychiatric nurses (especially doing Project 2000 and post-graduate courses), for psychologists and social workers (in training and in clinical practice), and for general practitioners finding themselves in the psychiatric front line.

We have been encouraged throughout the writing of the book by students and colleagues (at UCL Medical School and elsewhere) alike. We owe a particular debt of gratitude to those who have taken the time to criticize individual chapters: Profs Barnes and Dinan; Drs Alcorn, Allen, Appleby, Barnes, Bhugra, Chesser, Collis, Cookson, Dein, Eapen, Feinmann, Freeman, Gardner, Jackson, Kahle, Kennedy, Livingston, McCarthy, Norton, Read, Ring, Orrell, Stansfeld, Sturgeon and Tannock; Jamie Arkel, Gina Hossain, Cheryl Moore, Paul de Keyser and Pippa Vincent. The content has been much improved by their criticism, although responsibility for any errors remains, of course, our own. We hope that you, the reader, will also feel able to offer suggestions for improvements to future editions. We would also like to thank John Ludgate for his support and encouragement.

Finally, we owe an enormous debt of gratitude to Philippa Katona, the GP on the Clapham omnibus, who has offered inestimable tolerance and support during the many evenings of writing, and helped ensure that both text and diagrams were much more relevant and comprehensible than they would otherwise have been.

Cornelius Katona
Mary Robertson
London

1 The psychiatric history and mental state examination (MSE)

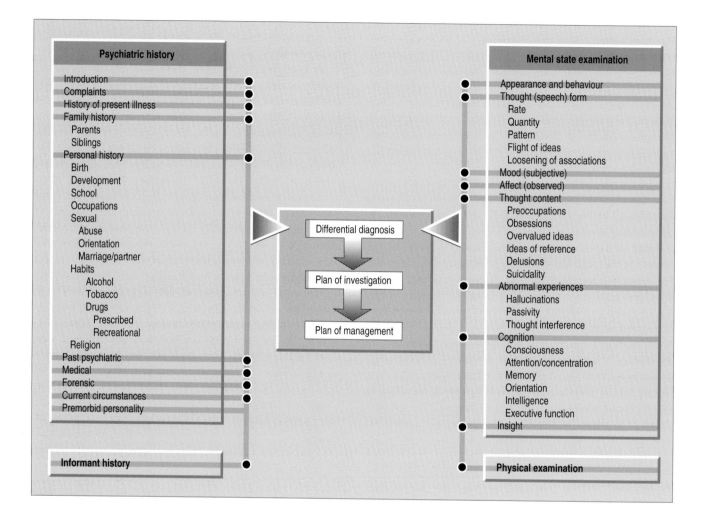

In taking a psychiatric history and assessing the mental state, it is crucial both to establish and maintain rapport and to be systematic in obtaining the necessary information. The outline below is intended as a schema for written documentation; greater flexibility is clearly required during the interview.

The psychiatric history

The history begins with an *introduction* noting the patient's name, age, marital status, occupation, ethnic origin, religion and circumstances of referral. Then follows the *complaint* (in the patient's own words) and the *history of the present illness* (duration, precipitating factors, effect on interpersonal relationships, working capacity and details of treatment to date). In the *family history*, note parents'/siblings' ages, occupations, physical and mental health and relationships with the patient. If a relative is deceased, note the cause of death and the patient's age at the time of death. Enquiry is made into family history of

psychiatric illness ('nervous breakdowns'), suicide, drug/alcohol abuse and forensic encounters.

The *personal history* begins with the patient's *early life and development* including details of the pregnancy (? planned) and birth (especially complications). Any serious illnesses, separations in childhood or delays in development are noted. The childhood home environment is described (geographical situation, atmosphere) as are details of school (academic achievements, relationships with peers, teachers). The occupational history is noted, listing jobs, reasons for change, work satisfaction, relationships with colleagues. Document details of sexual practices (past/present abuse, sexual orientation, difficulties, satisfaction), relationships, marriage (duration, details of partner, children) and, in the case of women, menstrual pattern, contraception, miscarriages, stillbirths and terminations of pregnancy.

Previous psychiatric history (dates of illnesses, symptoms, diagnoses, treatments, hospitalizations) and *past medical and surgical history* are obtained. The patient's alcohol, drug (prescribed and recreational) and tobacco *consumption* and any *forensic* history are recorded. The patient's attitude to and practice of religion, politics and hobbies are noted. The *premorbid personality* (e.g. character, social relations) and finally, details of the present circumstances (accommodation, occupation, financial details), are described.

The MSE

The patient's *appearance and behaviour* are documented, including general health, demeanour, manner, rapport, eye contact, degree of cooperation, cleanliness, clothing, self-care, facial expression, posture, motor activity, which may be excessive (agitation) or decreased (retardation), abnormal movements (tics, chorea, tremor, stereotypy (purposeless), mannerisms (goal-directed, understandable), gait abnormality or striking physical features.

Speech is described in terms of rate, quantity (increased = pressure (often with associated 'flight of ideas'); decreased = poverty), and pattern (spontaneity, coherence, rationality, directness (to the point or discursive) and perseveration (repeating words or topics)). Abnormal words (neologisms), puns or rhymes should be noted, giving verbatim examples if abnormal. Abnormal *form of thought* may be deduced, for example where connections between statements are difficult to follow ('loosening of associations'). The patient's subjective experience of thought may be abnormal as in thought block (thoughts disappear: 'my mind goes blank').

Changes in *mood and affect* are the commonest symptoms of psychiatric disorder, but also occur in physical illness and in healthy people at times of misfortune. *Mood* is subjective emotion as experienced by the individual, while *affect* is the observed (and often more transient) external manifestation of that emotion. Mood has been compared to climate, and affect to weather. Abnormalities of affect include blunting, lability, perplexity and suspiciousness. Abnormal mood states include depression, elation, euphoria (unconcerned contentment), anxiety and anger. It should be noted whether mood is consistent with thoughts and actions, or 'incongruous'.

Disorders of *thought content* include non-psychotic phenomena such as obsessional ideas (recurrent thoughts, feelings, images or impulses which are intrusive, persistent, senseless, unwelcome and recognized as the patient's own) and phobias (fear/anxiety which is out of proportion to the situation, cannot be reasoned or explained away and leads to avoidance behaviour). Suicidal ideation (thoughts) and intent (plans) are crucial.

Abnormal beliefs include overvalued ideas (abnormal beliefs or intense preoccupations, firmly held but comprehensible in the light of the subject's past experience and culturally shared belief systems). An example of this would be an intense but non-delusional feeling of guity responsibility following bereavement. Ideas of reference are when the patient feels that other people look at or talk about him/her because they notice things about him/her, but insight (see below) is retained. Delusions (fixed, false, firmly held beliefs out of keeping with the patient's culture, unaltered by evidence to the contrary, and for which the patient has no insight) may be primary (with no discernible connection with any previous experience or mood; autochthonous) or secondary (e.g. to mood). Passivity feelings are when the patient experiences outside control of or interference with his/her actions, feelings, perceptions and thoughts (thought interference). The latter may involve thought insertion or withdrawal (thoughts being put into and taken out of the person's mind) and thought broadcast (the experience that others can hear or read the individual's mind/thoughts).

Abnormal experiences include depersonalization, which is the unpleasant experience of subjective change, feeling detached, unreal, empty within, unable to feel emotion, watching oneself from outside, e.g. 'it feels as if I am cut off by a pane of glass'. The related phenomenon of derealization is the experience of the world or people in it seeming lifeless ('as if made out of cardboard').

Abnormalities of perception include illusions (distortions of perception of an external stimulus, e.g. interpreting a curtain cord as a snake); hallucinations (perceptions in the absence of an external stimulus which are experienced both as true and coming from the outside world); and pseudo-hallucinations (internal perceptions with preserved insight). Hallucinations can occur in any sensory modality, although auditory and visual are commonest. Some auditory hallucinations occur in normal individuals, when falling asleep (hypnagogic) or on waking (hypnopompic).

Within the *cognitive assessment*, the following are noted: level of consciousness, memory (long and short term, immediate recall), orientation in time (day, date, time), place, person, attention and concentration, general knowledge and intelligence. Educational background must be taken into account.

An assessment of the patient's *insight* (degree of correct understanding a patient has of his/her condition and its cause as well as his/her willingness to accept treatment) is made, after which the examiner notes his/her *reaction to the patient*.

The *physical examination* should focus on identifying (or excluding) conditions of which a suspicion has been raised in the history and MSE and/or with a known association with psychiatric illness.

In presenting a case, the history and MSE should be followed by a justified statement of diagnosis (or differential diagnosis), and concluded by a summary of possible aetiological factors (predisposing, precipitating and maintaining), and a plan for further investigation and management.

2 Diagnosis and classification in psychiatry

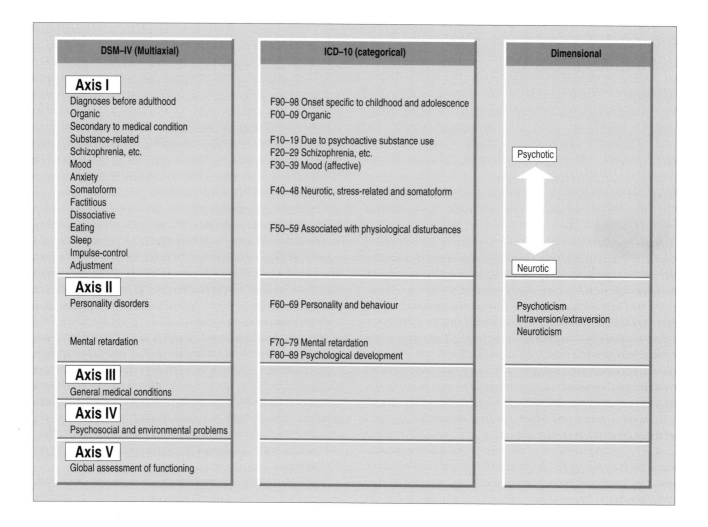

History

Diagnoses and classifications in psychiatry have undergone tremendous changes in the last 40 years. Before the 1950s, diagnoses were not only unreliable, but even had meanings that varied considerably across the world. By the end of that decade, 'antipsychiatrists' including Laing and Szasz had started to suggest that diagnoses and classification in psychiatry should be abandoned, together with the concept of mental illness. In the 1960s, the World Health Organization (WHO) instigated a world-wide programme (>30 countries) aimed at improving diagnosis and classification of mental disorders, fostering research into reliability of diagnosis and classification. The mental health section of the International Classification of Diseases (ICD) has subsequently been revised several times and is currently in its 10th edition (ICD-10). The American Psychiatric Association developed its own classificatory system, the Diagnostic and Statistical Manual of Mental Disorders (DSM); the current classification, DSM-IV, was published in 1994.

The concept of mental illness

Prior to considering the classification of mental illness, it is useful to note that, in general medicine, a distinction is made between 'disease' (objective physical pathology and known aetiology) and 'illness' (subjective distress). Most psychiatric conditions should not therefore be considered 'diseases' since in many the aetiology is 'multifactorial' and there is no demonstrable pathology. The advent of new techniques (e.g. neuroimaging) may, however, result in the emergence of definable psychiatric diseases. However, the concept of mental 'illness' is useful in defining a level of subjective distress greater in severity and/or duration than occurs in normal human experience. In addition, in the laws of many countries, psychiatrists need to diagnose 'mental illness' when certifying the need for compulsory admission to hospital and in 'forensic' (legal) psychiatry.

Aims and purposes

The purpose of classification in psychiatry, as in the rest of general medicine, is to identify groups of patients who are similar in their clinical features, course of disease, outcome and response to treatment, thus not only aiding individual clinical management but also providing patterns of treatment response and prognosis which can be extrapolated to future patients. A further purpose of classification of disease is to facilitate communication between professionals and research into the aetiology, prevention and treatment of psychiatric conditions. A final aim of classification is to improve the *reliability* (reproducibility between different settings) and *validity* (correctness) of diagnoses. Validity is more difficult to confirm but attempts have been made, including the examination of consistency of symptom patterns (statistical procedures such as 'cluster analysis' facilitate this) and demonstration of consistent treatment responses, long-term prognoses, genetic and biological correlates. *Discriminating symptoms* occur commonly in a defined syndrome, but rarely in other syndromes (e.g. thought broadcast/schizophrenia (see Chapter 3)), while *characteristic symptoms* occur frequently in the defined syndrome but also occur in other syndromes (e.g. depressed mood, which though common in depressive illness also occurs in schizophrenia, alcoholism, etc.). *Operational definitions* mean the specification of precise inclusion and exclusion criteria.

Types of classification

Traditionally, mental disorder is differentiated into *mental retardation* (learning disability, in which features of the disorder have been present from birth or an early age), *personality disorder* (usually present from childhood or adolescence onwards), *mental illness* (where there is an identifiable onset of illness preceded by normal functioning), *adjustment disorder* (less severe than mental illness, occuring in relation to stressful events or changed circumstances), *disorders of childhood* and *other disorders* (those which do not fit into any other group, including behavioural disorders and substance misuse). Mental illness has in turn traditionally been differentiated into *organic* and *functional (psychotic and neurotic)* types.

Three main ways of classifying include the *categorical, dimensional* and *multiaxial* types. *Categorical systems* describe a group of entirely separate conditions which are usually classified *hierarchically*, so that each patient can receive one main diagnosis (organic psychoses take precedence over functional psychoses which take precedence over neuroses). The terms *psychosis* (with hallucinations and delusions, lacking insight (see Chapter 1) and a more severe form of illness) and *neurosis* (mental distress in the absence of hallucinations or delusions, insight retained and less severe illness) are widely used and may be regarded as a categorical system. Within this system most depressive and anxiety disorders would fall within the neurotic category. *Dimensional systems* use a *continuum* rather than categories and have been used mainly to classify personality. For example, Hans Eysenck has proposed three dimensions of personality: introversion/extraversion, neuroticism and psychoticism. A psychotic/neurotic continuum for major mental illness has been suggested by Kendell. Finally, *multiaxial systems* categorize the patient on *several axes*, rating patients on several separate categorical systems each measuring a different aspect (e.g. psychiatric diagnosis, personality, intelligence).

Systems of classification

The two main current systems of classification include the *ICD* and the *DSM*. ICD-10 is an *uniaxial system* which attempts to standardize using *descriptive definitions* of the syndromes and operational criteria, as well as producing directives on differential diagnosis. DSM-IV, a *multiaxial* system, relies on operational criteria (rather than descriptive definitions). It states which symptoms need to be present (often quantifying their number and requiring a specific length of time for symptoms to be present) as well as exclusion criteria. DSM-IV includes the following: axis I = clinical syndromes and other conditions that may be a focus of clinical attention; axis II = personality disorders and mental retardation (the latter classified by severity rather than aetiology); axis III = general medical conditions; axis IV = psychosocial and environmental problems; axis V = global assessment of functioning. ICD-10, in contrast, is more reliant on clinical description, although a research supplement has been produced which provides operational criteria more similar to those of DSM-IV.

ICD-10 and DSM-IV use broadly matching, although not always identical, major diagnostic categories as follows.

1 Disorders Usually First Diagnosed in Infancy, Childhood or Adolescence (which may reflect developmental disorders, discrete illnesses or a combination of the two).

2 Delirium, Dementia, Amnestic and other Cognitive Disorders.

3 Mental Disorders Due to a General Medical Condition Not Elsewhere Classified.

4 Psychoactive Substance-Related Disorders.

5 Schizophrenia (including Schizotypal, Delusional and other Psychotic Disorders).

6 Mood (affective) Disorders.

7 Anxiety (neurotic) Disorders.

8 Somatoform, Factitious and Dissociative Disorders.

9 Sexual and Identity Disorders.

10 Eating Disorders.

11 Sleep Disorders.

12 Impulse-Control Disorders.

13 Adjustment Disorders.

3 Schizophrenia: phenomenology and aetiology

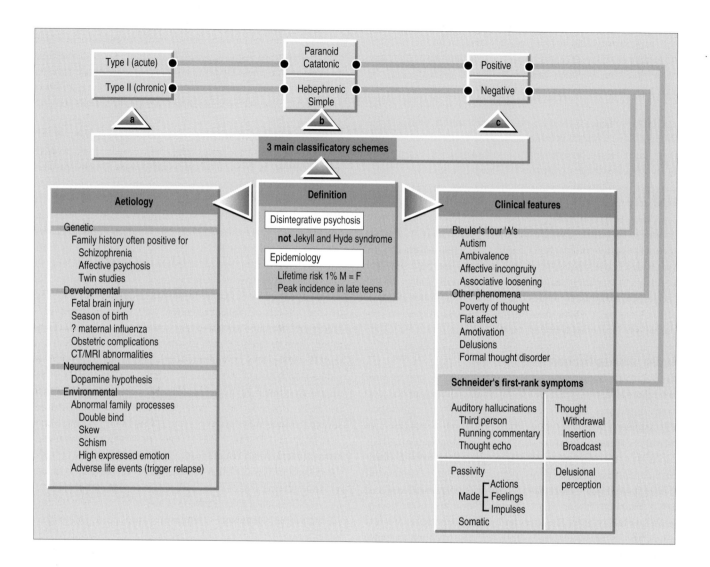

Introduction, history and definition

Many lay people misconceive schizophrenia as a 'split personality' or 'Jekyll and Hyde' phenomenon in which the individual can behave quite normally at times but is liable to change suddenly and become bizarre or dangerous. In fact, schizophrenia (literally 'split mind') is a disintegrative psychosis, characterized by 'splitting' of normal links between perception, mood, thinking, behaviour and contact with reality. This results in delusions (fixed, false, unshakable beliefs), hallucinations (perceptions without stimuli, e.g. hearing voices), disorganized thinking/speech (e.g. incoherence) and behaviour, negative symptoms (e.g. affective flattening) and social and/or occupational dysfunction. Emil Kraepelin (1893) suggested the distinction between the organic psychoses (where a physiological disturbance could be shown, e.g. infection) and functional psychoses (with no such changes), and as an example of the latter,

coined the term 'dementia praecox' (characterized by irreversible deterioration of mental functions, e.g. withdrawal, self-neglect and bizarre behaviour). This corresponds broadly to current concepts of schizophrenia.

Classification

There are three main classificatory systems. Crow suggested *type I* (*acute* onset, positive symptoms (hallucinations, delusions), normal brain ventricular size, good prognosis, good response to neuroleptics, dopamine abnormalities) and *type II* (*chronic*, negative symptoms (e.g. flat affect) enlarged ventricles, poor prognosis, poor response to neuroleptics, neurone loss). Another system suggests four types: *paranoid* (delusions, auditory hallucinations); *catatonic* (motor immobility (e.g. stupor), excessive activity (excitement)), rigidity, posturing (e.g. waxy flexibility = maintaining strange postures), echolalia (copying speech), echopraxia (copying behaviours)); **hebephrenic (disorganized)** (early onset, thought incoherence, disorganized behaviour, blunted or incongruous affect); and **simple** (deterioration, defect state). Andreasen suggested **positive** (hallucinations, delusions) and **negative** (poverty of speech, flat affect, avolition (poor motivation), poor attention) types. There are overlaps between these typologies and, in any case, few patients fit neatly into one type only.

Epidemiology

Schizophrenia occurs in 15–20/100 000 individuals per year, with a lifetime morbidity risk of 0.85% (M = F) and a peak incidence in late teens or early adulthood.

Clinical features

Classic symptoms include **Bleuler's four 'A's**: **A**utism (withdrawal from reality into an inner fantasy world), **A**mbivalence (coexistence of conflicting ideas, feelings), **A**ffective incongruity (affect and thoughts disassociated (e.g. smiling when discussing something sad) or blunting (flat)), and **A**ssociative loosening ('thought disorder', i.e. loosening of logical connections between thoughts).

Schneider's First-Rank Symptoms (SFRS) include specific types of auditory hallucination (third person discussing the patient, making a running commentary on the patient); thought echo (hearing one's own thoughts out loud (*echo de la pensée*)); thought withdrawal (thoughts taken out of head); thought insertion (thoughts put into mind); thought broadcast (thoughts available to others; the patient thinking everyone is thinking in unison with him/her); passivity (made acts, feelings, impulses, i.e. being controlled by outside forces); somatic passivity (bodily sensations controlled from without, e.g. blood boils after being struck by lightning); and delusional (apophanous) perception (attribution of a new meaning (with delusional intensity), usually self-referential, to a normally perceived object and often preceded by delusional mood (altered affect of fear, e.g. 'I heard a police siren and knew I had been appointed one of God's prophets', perplexity, foreboding, ecstasy, 'something going on around me')). Schneider considered SFRS diagnostic of acute schizophrenia if organic conditions were excluded. In fact, 8% of patients with non-schizophrenic functional psychoses have one or more SFRS, and 20% of people with chronic schizophrenia never show them. Second-rank symptoms, which are less diagnostically specific, include catatonic behaviour, secondary delusions and other hallucinations.

Other characteristic features of schizophrenia include poverty of thought (decreased thoughts and speech), flat (blunted) or incongruous affect, amotivation and delusions (often bizarre).

Formal thought disorder (e.g. loosening of associations, i.e. getting off the bus is successful because coffee is best), 'Knight's move thinking' (wandering off the point), neologisms (new words, or ordinary words used in a special way), concrete thinking (inability to deal with abstract ideas) and word salad (jumbled nonsense), are all found in schizophrenia.

Delusions may be primary (arising *de novo*, e.g. 'I am God') or secondary (arising from another morbid experience, e.g. hallucinations, passivity or mood). The content of delusions is dependent on social and cultural backgrounds (e.g. religious persons believing they are God, doctor believing X-rays are being beamed into his/her house by the neighbours). Delusions in schizophrenia are usually systematized and often bizarre. Content is frequently persecutory (some individual or group is out to harm them, e.g. by poisoning), or of reference (e.g. patient is mentioned on TV news or knows that people are talking about him/her). It is customary (but incorrect) for English-speaking psychiatrists to use the term 'paranoid' instead of persecutory. Delusions may be of marital infidelity (incorrect beliefs of partner being unfaithful), grandiosity (patients believing they are God, Monarch, Napoleon), or nihilism.

Both DSM-IV and ICD-10 have **operational criteria** for schizophrenia which specify the presence of specific symptoms for certain lengths of time, and exclude other major disorders (e.g. depression).

Aetiology

There is a strong suggestion of **genetic factors** as aetiologically significant in schizophrenia, with a positive **family history** of schizophrenia and affective psychoses being reported with increased frequency in relatives of schizophrenics. **Twin studies** indicate that concordance rates are higher in monozygotic than dizygotic twins (MZ/DZ = 42 : 9%). **Adoptive studies** show that adopted-away offspring of schizophrenics have an increased (about 12%) chance of developing schizophrenia. No gene has yet been identified. **Developmental** problems have also been invoked as aetiological, with fetal 'brain injury' (seasonality of birth (more births in winter)), low birth weight, order in large families, possibly maternal influenza during pregnancy, increased obstetric complications and perinatal injuries being suggested; computerized brain tomographic (CT) and magnetic resonance imaging (MRI) scans show increased ventricular size (in type I schizophrenia). 'Soft' neurological signs (e.g. abnormal movements, left-handedness) and temporal lobe epilepsy are associated with schizophrenia. The **dopamine hypothesis** of schizophrenia suggests dopamine excess or overactivity in mesolimbic pathways (amphetamines release dopamine and lead to psychosis; antipsychotics, which block dopamine receptors, treat psychosis successfully); increased dopamine receptors have been found at post-mortem. **Abnormal family processes** have been invoked but not established as aetiologically significant. These include double-bind (parents convey two or more conflicting, incompatible messages at same time), skew (overprotective, intrusive, dominant mother; oversubmissive father), schism (hostility between parents), high expressed emotion (EE, relatives overinvolved or making excessive critical comments). People with schizophrenia experience an excess of **life events** in the 3 weeks before the onset of acute symptoms.

4 Schizophrenia: management and prognosis

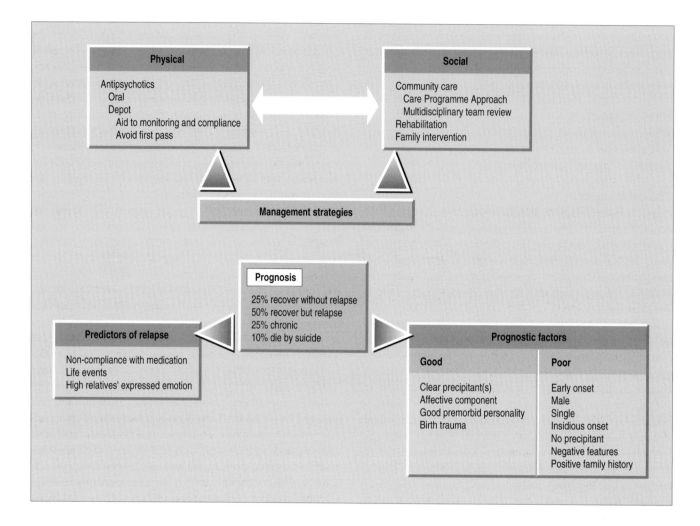

Physical	
Antipsychotics	
Oral	
Depot	
Aid to monitoring and compliance	
Avoid first pass	

Social
Community care
Care Programme Approach
Multidisciplinary team review
Rehabilitation
Family intervention

Management strategies

Prognosis

25% recover without relapse
50% recover but relapse
25% chronic
10% die by suicide

Predictors of relapse

Non-compliance with medication
Life events
High relatives' expressed emotion

Prognostic factors

Good	Poor
Clear precipitant(s)	Early onset
Affective component	Male
Good premorbid personality	Single
Birth trauma	Insidious onset
	No precipitant
	Negative features
	Positive family history

Management

Management includes ***antipsychotic (neuroleptic)*** medications (see pp. 72–73) and ***psychosocial interventions***. Ideally, if the patient is in a first episode and/or requiring supervision, treatment should be as an ***in-patient*** in a psychiatric hospital either informally (if patient agrees), or under a 'Section' of the Mental Health Act if necessary (see pp. 62–63). Admission not only prevents the consequences of disordered behaviour and reduces the effects of psychosocial precipitants, e.g. family conflict, but also allows treatment (e.g. medication) to be initiated under supervision. In addition, patients with schizophrenia often lack family support and thus require admission, which may itself be therapeutic.

Antipsychotics are the drugs of choice. There is good evidence that they not only tranquillize and sedate the patient (non-specifically), but also have a specific therapeutic effect on the 'positive symptoms' in the acute episode (e.g. hallucinations, delusions, passivity phenomena, thought alienation). 'Typical'

antipsychotics may, however, neither improve negative symptoms nor prevent deterioration. If the patient is agitated, overactive or violent, he/she may require sedation (e.g. with chlorpromazine). 'Atypical' antipsychotics (see pp. 72–73), may be effective in treating 'negative' as well as 'positive' symptoms. Medication may be administered ***orally, intramuscularly*** or by long-acting ***depot injections*** (e.g. flupenthixol (Depixol); fluphenazine (Modecate)), which provide long-term prophylaxis, increase compliance, allow regular contact with either community psychiatric nurses (CPNs) or clinics and avoid first pass metabolism. 'Depot groups' may facilitate monitoring and encourage compliance through peer pressure.

If the patient experiences extrapyramidal side-effects (e.g. dystonia, oculogyric crisis), anticholinergic drugs (e.g. procyclidine, benztropine) should be given immediately to reduce the extrapyramidal side-effects, making the patient more comfortable and rendering the antipsychotics more 'acceptable'. Regular antiparkinsonian drugs should be avoided as they have unwanted side-effects (e.g. blurred vision, dry mouth), may be abused, may worsen or provoke tardive dyskinesia (TD) and, in excess, may cause excitement and confusion. TD may respond to reduction/cessation of antipsychotics or to tetrabenazine but is irreversible in up to 50% of cases. People with schizophrenia can become depressed and may require antidepressant medication. Occasionally, *electroconvulsive therapy (ECT)* may be useful (e.g. catatonic stupor, excitement). After discharge from hospital, regular out-patient appointments are an important support as well as a facility for monitoring the patient's mental state and medication.

Psychotherapy (supportive) and counselling are important for all patients with schizophrenia and for their families and/or carers. Cognitive-behavioural techniques may be useful in helping patients cope with persistent delusions and hallucinations, and in rewarding appropriate behaviour patterns. Such techniques are particularly useful in more chronic, potentially institutionalized patients. Operant techniques may be helpful in patients with socially embarrassing or withdrawn behaviour. Family therapy helps the family reduce their excessive 'expressed emotion' (EE) or deal with separation from the patient. Psychoanalysis is not only not helpful but may even be harmful.

Rehabilitation is an important part of treatment, and usually includes occupational therapy, counselling and supportive psychotherapy while in hospital. Social workers may also help with sorting out accommodation, finances, etc. (troubles which may adversely affect the patient's mental state). Institutionalization (with the handicaps it brings) must be avoided; therefore the patient should be encouraged to go on leave from hospital, have retraining in skills and employment and be discharged as soon as is practical. After discharge, further rehabilitation can take place at day hospitals, half-way houses, sheltered workshops and/or day centres. These are important for ensuring medication, providing recreation, activities and appropriate work-experience. Both under- and overstimulation must be avoided.

It is important to note that a combination of antipsychotic medication, supportive psychotherapy and social measures is more efficacious than medication alone.

Community care is becomingly increasingly important with the closing down of the large psychiatric hospitals in many parts of the world. Appropriate accommodation is important, and there may be fine balance between independence and potential isolation; hostels or half-way houses are a good compromise. A concern about community care is that, in many parts of the world, it is being implemented without adequate financial and personnel resources; the more disadvantaged patients may well, in these instances, become vagrants or be imprisoned. Recent tragedies in the UK and other parts of the world have attracted media and government attention and resulted in new measures and legislations to deal with the problems of 'at risk' (e.g. of violence or suicide) in the community. The Care Programme Approach (CPA) in the UK emphasizes multidisciplinary team (MDT) work and regular patient review. Under the CPA, each patient is assigned a designated 'key worker' who may be any member of the MDT, such as the CPN or community psychiatric occupational therapist. This 'key worker' will visit the discharged patient, providing support, monitoring the mental state and treatment compliance, and helping with practical aspects of daily life (e.g. sorting out finances). Individuals at serious risk of suicide, self-neglect or serious violence, may be placed on a supervision register and followed up very closely by 'key workers' who may instigate admission if the individual deteriorates sufficiently to cause concern.

Prognosis

One-quarter of patients with schizophrenia recover without a subsequent relapse, 50% recover but relapse in the future (often with increasingly severe residual symptoms) and 25% fail to recover at all, developing a chronic illness: 10% die by suicide. Suicide risk is more in young males with persistent hallucinations or delusions, especially just before/during the first 3 months after discharge. Better prognosis is encountered in the developing world, which may be due to the social structure, family support or less stigma.

Good prognostic factors include a clear precipitant prior to the onset of the schizophrenic episode, older age at onset, an acute onset, 'positive' symptoms, a strong affective component (e.g. depressed), paranoid subtype, good premorbid personality, history of birth trauma, higher intelligence and a normal CT scan. Prognosis is also better with 'atypical' cases, e.g. schizo-affective disorder (illness typical of schizophrenia but with either a major depressive, manic or mixed episode, concurrent with symptoms of schizophrenia).

Poor prognostic factors include male gender, being single, social isolation, an insidious early onset without precipitants, hebephrenic symptomatology, negative features (e.g. amotivation), lack of affective component (flat, blunted affect), low IQ, low social class, abnormal premorbid personality and a positive family history of schizophrenia.

Factors that predict relapse include non-compliance with antipsychotic medication, adverse 'life events' (e.g. death of close relative) and high EE (critical comments or overinvolvement in the family, measured during a standardized research interview), if contact is experienced for over 35 hours a week.

5 Depression

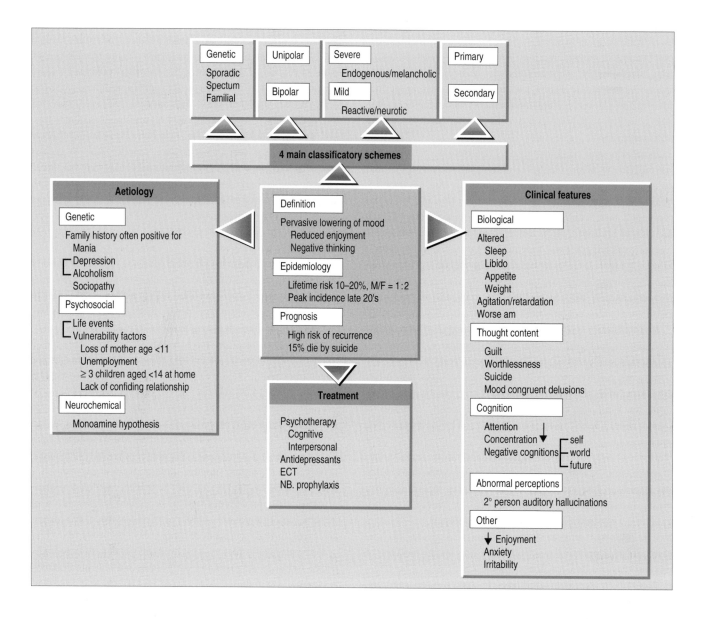

Definitions and classification

Depression is primarily a disorder of emotion; its essential feature is a pervasive lowering of mood. Most patients also have a reduced level of enjoyment (anhedonia) and negative patterns of thinking. There is, however, wide variation in symptomatology and in severity. This has resulted in considerable disagreement as to classification. Four main schemes have emerged. The best known of these proposes a dichotomy between 'endogenous' and 'neurotic' (also termed 'reactive') depression. The former is more severe, less likely to have external precipitants, and is characterized by prominent 'biological' features (see below), whereas the latter is milder, more understandable in terms of external circumstances, more heterogeneous and may show symptomatic overlap with anxiety. In recent years the notion of a mild/severe continuum has largely replaced the 'endogenous'/ 'neurotic' dichotomy. Depressions may also be seen as bipolar (having a tendency to abnormal upswings as well as downswings of mood) vs. unipolar (episodes of depression only); and secondary (associated with other psychiatric or physical illness) vs. primary. The fourth classification is genetic, dividing depressions into 'familial' (positive family history of depression); 'spectrum' (positive family history of related conditions such as alcoholism and personality disorders) and 'sporadic' (no relevant family history).

The unipolar/bipolar and severe/mild distinctions are favoured in the current ICD-10 and DSM-IV classifications (see pp. 10–11).

Clinical features

Depression manifests with alterations of biological function and of cognition as well as of mood. Anxiety or irritability may predominate over depressed mood. The main biological changes involve sleep, appetite and libido. In 'endogenous' depression, sleep is reduced with a pattern of early waking and maximal lowering of mood in the morning (diurnal variation). Appetite is reduced with associated weight loss and, in severe cases, reluctance or refusal even to drink. Libido is reduced or absent. Anhedonia is accompanied by loss of motivation. Motor activity is often altered, with retardation (of speech and/or movement), agitation or both. In 'neurotic' depressions the pattern may be inverted with initial anxiety-related insomnia, subsequent over-sleeping and increased appetite.

Thought content often includes negative, pessimistic thoughts about the self, the world and the future (Beck's cognitive triad), thoughts of death or suicide and feelings of guilt and worthlessness. Cognitive function may be impaired, with reduced attention and/or concentration. Delusions and hallucinations are usually 'mood congruent'. The former typically concern illness or death. The latter are relatively rare, usually auditory in the second person and accusing, condemning or urging suicide.

Differential diagnosis

Depression may be difficult to distinguish from normal sadness, particularly in the context of bereavement (see Chapter 8) or severe physical illness. The diagnosis depends on finding a pattern of characteristic features (as above) accompanying the low mood; and on the degree and duration of associated disability. Predominant anxiety symptoms may obscure the diagnosis of depression. Depressive retardation may be difficult to distinguish from the affective flattening of schizophrenia.

Epidemiology

The lifetime risk of depression is about 10%, with rates almost doubled in women. First onset is typically in the third decade (earlier for bipolar disorder) with point prevalence higher in middle and old age. Depression is commoner in urban than in rural areas, and, particularly in women, in the working classes.

Aetiology

A genetic contribution is evident in both twin and adoption studies, less markedly for unipolar than bipolar depression. Neurochemical and neuroendocrine mechanisms have been proposed. The dominant neurochemical theory is the 'monoamine hypothesis' based on the observations (in the 1960s) that monoamine (particularly noradrenaline and serotonin) metabolites in cerebrospinal fluid (CSF) and urine are reduced in depressed patients, and that antidepressants increase monoamine availability. This has been modified to emphasize changes in monoamine neuroreceptors (particularly betaadrenoreceptors and $5HT_2$ receptors) related to depression and to antidepressant treatment. Neuroendocrine abnormalities found in some depressed patients include hypercortisolaemia (and related impairment of dexamethasone-induced suppression of cortisol secretion), and impaired thyroid axis activity. Depression is also associated with characteristic sleep-EEG changes, and reduced frontal lobe blood flow.

The most important exogenous factors implicated are recent adverse life events (such as bereavement and deteriorating physical health), and parental loss and/or major stress or abuse in childhood (which appears to increase vulnerability to depression in response to life events). These factors may be involved in endogenous as well as neurotic depression. Adverse current social circumstances, especially unemployment and lack of a confiding relationship, may also increase such vulnerability. Several physical illnesses (most endocrine disorders, many cancers, some viral infections) are specifically associated with depression. Women appear particularly vulnerable to episodes of depression in the weeks following childbirth.

Management

Most depressive illnesses can be managed in the primary care setting, although many are undetected. Detection rates can be enhanced by remembering that depressed patients often present with other conditions, and/or by simple screening questionnaires. Management starts with risk assessment, in terms of self-neglect and, most importantly, suicide. Psychiatric referral is indicated if suicide risk is high, or if the depression is severe, unresponsive to initial treatment or recurrent. Physical treatments (see Chapter 33) include tricyclic and newer antidepressants (e.g. selective serotonin reuptake inhibitors (SSRIs)) and can have a 60–70% response rate but frequently fail because of inadequate dosage, duration or compliance. ECT is very effective in severe cases, particularly where delusions and/or retardation are present. Refractory depression may respond to combination treatments such as lithium augmentation. Specific psychological techniques (including cognitive–behaviour therapy (CBT), interpersonal and problem-solving psychotherapy) have similar success rates to antidepressants in non-psychotic depression; CBT also has some prophylactic effect. Continuing antidepressants for at least 6 months after a first episode reduces relapse rate; in recurrent depression prophylactic effects have been demonstrated for up to 5 years.

Prognosis

Single episodes of depression usually last between 3 and 8 months; about 20% of patients remain depressed for 2 years or more. About 50% have recurrences; this rises to 80% in severe cases (such as those requiring in-patient care). Recurrent episodes tend to become increasingly severe with shortening of disease-free periods, emphasizing the importance of prophylactic treatment. Lifetime suicide risk is 15% in severe depression but much lower in milder illness. Predictors of poor outcome include early onset, initial symptom severity and psychiatric or physical comorbidity.

6 Bipolar affective disorder (including mania)

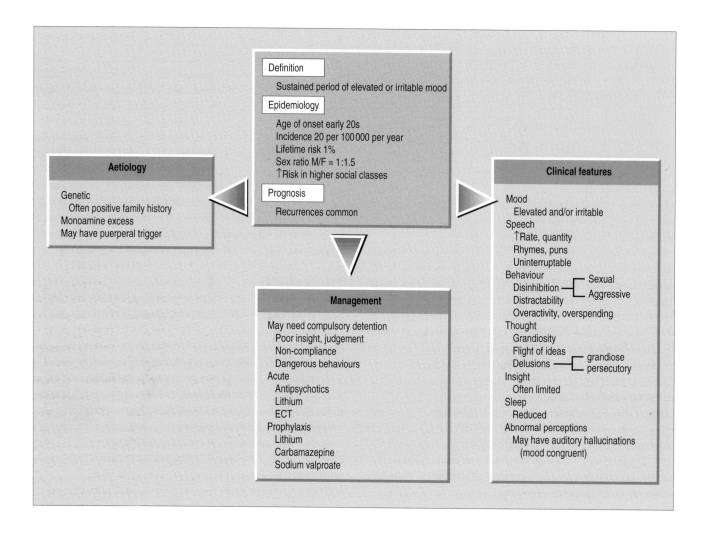

Definitions and classification

The bipolar affective disorders are characterized by recurrent episodes of altered mood and activity, involving up- as well as down-swings. Recent classificatory systems (DSM-IV, ICD-10) have therefore had to define both individual episodes and patterns of recurrence. Individual episodes include major depressive episode (described in the chapter on depressive disorders); manic episode; hypomanic episode (less severe); and mixed episode, in which features of mania and major depression alternate rapidly. Patterns of recurrence can be classified as Bipolar I Disorder (with one or more manic or mixed episodes and, usually, one or more major depressive episodes); Bipolar II Disorder (recurrent major depressive and hypomanic but not manic episodes); and Cyclothymic Disorder, with chronic mood fluctuations over at least 2 years including individual episodes of hypomania (but not mania) and of depression insufficient in severity to meet major depression criteria.

Clinical features

The cardinal clinical feature of a manic episode is alteration in mood which is often elated and expansive but may also be characterized by intense irritability. Associated features include increased psychomotor activity (rapid thinking and speech, distractibility, decreased need for sleep); decreased social inhibition and disregard for potentially painful consequences (sexual overactivity, overspending, indulgence in poorly considered or inappropriate business, religious or political initiatives); and exaggerated optimism and inflated self-esteem, which may be reflected in grandiose delusions or hallucinations. Mood incongruent psychotic features may also be found; indeed, one or more Schneiderian first-rank symptoms (see Chapter 3) are occasionally present but may indicate a schizo-affective disorder. Heightened sensory awareness is common. More specific speech abnormalities include uninterruptibility and sound- rather than sense-triggered speech content (punning, clanging).

Insight is often variable or absent. Manic and hypomanic episodes are distinguished on the basis that mania is more severe (causing marked work, social and/or interpersonal disruption) and usually necessitates hospitalization, whereas hypomania is less severe and disruptive and fewer clinical features are present.

Differential diagnosis

The most important differential diagnoses are organic. These include substance abuse (particularly amphetamines or cocaine) and mood abnormalities secondary to endocrine disturbance (idiopathic Cushing's syndrome or steroid-induced psychoses) or epilepsy. 'Secondary' mania, or organic mood disorder may also be precipitated by severe physical illness (particularly stroke). Acute schizophrenia may present very much like mania: persecutory delusions are common in both, and the distinction between formal thought disorder and flight of ideas may be difficult. Other conditions to consider include attention-deficit hyperactivity disorder and transient psychoses induced by extreme stress. In both of these, elevation of mood is rare.

Epidemiology

The lifetime prevalence of bipolar disorder is about 1%, with a ratio of bipolar I/cyclothymia/bipolar II of about 2 : 2 : 1. The female/male ratio is about 1.5 : 1, the female excess being in the bipolar II group. Peak age of first onset is in the early 20s. Several studies have shown higher prevalence rates in higher social classes, probably reflecting differences in access to diagnosis and treatment.

Aetiology

There is clear evidence of a strong familial component. Rates of both bipolar disorder (including cyclothymia) and unipolar depression are commoner than expected in first-degree relatives of bipolar subjects. Both sex-linked and autosomal inheritance have been proposed. A number of neuroendocrine abnormalities have been described including hypercortisolaemia, increased aldosterone secretion and blunted growth hormone response to hypoglycaemia. The findings are less consistent than in depressive illness, and usually similar rather than opposite. Some studies suggest that manic episodes may be precipitated by severe stress. In particular, there is a markedly increased risk of manic episodes occurring in the early postpartum weeks; this may relate to dopamine receptor supersensitivity associated with precipitate postpartum falls in oestrogen and progesterone levels. Psychodynamic models of mania implicate denial of loss or loss-associated conflict in order to avoid depression, and/or loss of superego ('conscience') control.

Management

Acute mania almost invariably requires hospitalization. Since patients often lose insight early, this may require detention without consent, using appropriate mental health legislation. Exclusion of organic causes is vital. Antipsychotics (in similar dosage to that used in schizophrenia) form the mainstay of acute management of both mania and hypomania. Antipsychotics are effective both in controlling overactivity and agitation, and (somewhat more slowly) in reducing elation and disinhibition. Lorazepam may be useful for rapid tranquillization Lithium is also effective as an acute antimanic agent, although it lacks the potential for very rapid behavioural control. In patients unresponsive to antipsychotics (particularly where extreme overactivity is a threat to physical health), ECT may be effective. Maintenance treatment with lithium has been shown in many controlled trials to reduce the frequency and severity of subsequent episodes; its 'real-life' effectiveness is harder to demonstrate and probably depends on careful supervision and education enabling good compliance. Lithium therapy (which may also be useful in cyclothymia) requires comprehensive pre-initiation screening (including renal and thyroid function estimation) and regular monitoring in view both of its narrow therapeutic range and its long-term potential to induce hypothyroidism. A number of anticonvulsants (carbamazepine, sodium valproate and possibly lamotrigine) appear to be effective in preventing manic relapse, particularly where psychotic feelings have been prominent. Psychotherapeutic support is important in helping patients come to terms with their illness and their remorse at their past manic behaviour.

Prognosis

The lifetime prognosis following a single manic episode is poor, with 90% of patients having manic and/or depressive recurrences (averaging four episodes in 10 years). In bipolar I disorder, both frequency and severity of episodes tend to increase for the first four or five episodes, but tend subsequently to plateau. Long-term functional prognosis (work, family, etc.) is almost as poor as in schizophrenia. A minority develop 'rapid cycling' with four or more episodes a year; they have a particularly poor prognosis and seldom respond to lithium. There is an overall increase in premature mortality, only partially explained by a suicide rate of 10%. Successful lithium prophylaxis (reflecting self-selection for good prognosis as well as good response to lithium) not only modifies severity and duration of episodes, but appears to reduce both suicide and overall mortality. Prognosis for Bipolar II disorder is better, although there remains a high suicide risk. Cyclothymia has a chronic course and an approximately 30% risk of developing full-blown bipolar disorder.

7 Suicide and deliberate self-harm (DSH)

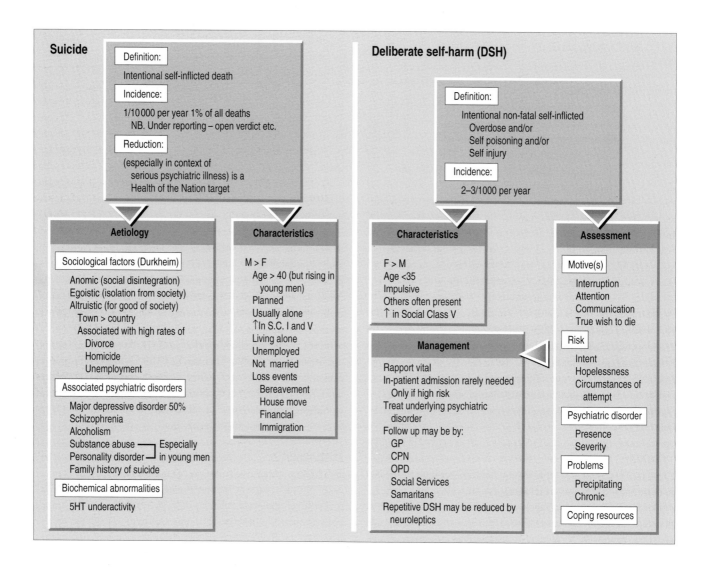

Suicide

Definition:
Intentional self-inflicted death

Incidence:
1/10 000 per year 1% of all deaths
NB. Under reporting – open verdict etc.

Reduction:
(especially in context of
serious psychiatric illness) is a
Health of the Nation target

Aetiology

Sociological factors (Durkheim)
Anomic (social disintegration)
Egoistic (isolation from society)
Altruistic (for good of society)
Town > country
Associated with high rates of
Divorce
Homicide
Unemployment

Associated psychiatric disorders
Major depressive disorder 50%
Schizophrenia
Alcoholism
Substance abuse ⎤ Especially
Personality disorder ⎦ in young men
Family history of suicide

Biochemical abnormalities
5HT underactivity

Characteristics

M > F
Age > 40 (but rising in
  young men)
Planned
Usually alone
↑In S.C. I and V
Living alone
Unemployed
Not married
Loss events
  Bereavement
  House move
  Financial
  Immigration

Deliberate self-harm (DSH)

Definition:
Intentional non-fatal self-inflicted
Overdose and/or
Self poisoning and/or
Self injury

Incidence:
2–3/1000 per year

Characteristics

F > M
Age <35
Impulsive
Others often present
↑ in Social Class V

Management

Rapport vital
In-patient admission rarely needed
  Only if high risk
Treat underlying psychiatric
  disorder
Follow up may be by:
  GP
  CPN
  OPD
  Social Services
  Samaritans
Repetitive DSH may be reduced by
  neuroleptics

Assessment

Motive(s)
Interruption
Attention
Communication
True wish to die

Risk
Intent
Hopelessness
Circumstances of
  attempt

Psychiatric disorder
Presence
Severity

Problems
Precipitating
Chronic

Coping resources

The assessment and acute management of DSH is probably the most critical psychiatric task facing the non-psychiatrist—particularly the (relatively inexperienced) medical houseman or casualty officer. Recognition of suicide risk is, together with better detection and management of psychiatric illness as a whole, crucial in reducing the suicide rate which, in the UK, has been identified as a National Health target.

Definitions
Suicide may be defined as intentional self-inflicted death; DSH represents intentionally self-inflicted harm without a fatal outcome.

Suicide
Epidemiology
International suicide rates vary widely, with the highest incidence in Hungary, the former Soviet Union and Finland. There are about 5000 suicides/year in England and Wales, an annual incidence of approximately 1/10 000 and representing about 1% of all deaths. Suicide rates in the UK are about three times higher in men than in women. Suicide rates in young men have recently risen sharply in most developed countries; highest rates are nonetheless found in the elderly.

Aetiology
Factors implicated in the aetiology of suicide can be classified as social, biological and psychiatric. Durkheim's social model described two main types of suicide: anomic and egoistic. Anomic suicide reflects a society's disintegration and loss of shared values; this is reflected in positive correlations between rates of suicide and of unemployment and homicide, reductions in suicide rate in wartime (social unity in adversity) and in Roman Catholic countries, and in the higher suicide rates in

urban than rural communities. The relationship between suicide and unemployment is also found at individual level, with job loss in men being associated with increased suicide risk both in themselves and their spouses. Some of this association is, however, explained by the increased risk of unemployment in the mentally ill. Egoistic suicide involves individuals' separation from otherwise cohesive social groups and finds some reflection in the higher suicide rates following bereavement and moving house, in immigrants, in people living alone, and divorced or single, compared to people who are married. A further social factor is availability of means: high rates in the USA have been linked to ease of obtaining firearms; UK rates fell sharply when toxic coal gas was replaced by (relatively) harmless natural gas. A positive family history of suicide is associated with increased suicide risk. A large proportion of completed suicides have consulted their general practitioners in the weeks prior to suicide, highlighting the need to recognize people at risk and consequent prevention. Although no consistent biological correlate of suicide has been found, evidence both from brain and CSF studies in suicides and suicide attempters (particularly those using violent means) suggests that serotonergic underactivity (as reflected in levels of 5HT and its metabolites, as well as in 5HT receptors and uptake sites) may be involved.

Perhaps the strongest association with suicide is psychiatric illness, with rates increased 50-fold in psychiatric in-patients, and retrospective 'psychiatric autopsy' studies suggesting that a specific psychiatric diagnosis can be made in almost all suicides. Specific diagnoses implicated include major depression (with a lifetime suicide risk of 15%), schizophrenia (10%), alcoholism (3–4%), and (less consistently) personality disorder (present in 30–60% of completed suicides), anorexia nervosa, substance misuse and obsessive–compulsive disorder (OCD). The relationship between depression and suicide is strongest in old age. In contrast, the recent increase in suicide rates in young men is associated with personality disorders and substance abuse. Suicide rates are also increased in people with chronic painful illnesses.

The acronym 'SAD PERSONS' is an *aide memoire* for risk factors in suicides: **S**ex, **A**ge, **D**epression, **P**revious attempts, **E**thanol abuse, **R**ational thinking loss (particularly psychosis), **S**ocial support lacking, **O**rganised plan, **N**o pastimes and **S**ickness (with special attention to medical disorders that have been shown to increase risk).

DSH

Epidemiology and correlates
DSH is a much commoner event than completed suicide, with an annual incidence of 2–3/1000 in the UK, where (in contrast to the USA) most cases involve drug overdose rather than physical self-injury. Unlike completed suicide, DSH is commoner in women and the under 35s. DSH is commoner in lower social classes and in the single and divorced. Like suicide, DSH is associated with psychiatric illness, particularly depression (usually mild) and personality disorder.

Assessment
The immediate priority is medical stabilization. Subsequent psychiatric assessment involves establishing a rapport (essential if the DSH is to be a springboard to appropriate management) and necessitating a suspension of the assessor's pejorative judgements. Relevant interview topics include identification of motive(s), acute and chronic problems and associated coping strategies, and of current psychiatric illness. DSH is often precipitated by undesirable life events. In most cases, its motive can be understood in terms of one or more of a desire to *interrupt* a sequence of events seen as both inevitable and undesirable; a need for *attention* or to *communicate* (decoding and transmission of such communications may itself be effective in reducing subsequent risk); and a true *wish to die*. The latter, although probably the single best indicator of high subsequent risk of suicide, is seldom either unequivocal or stable. Subjects at high risk have a clinical profile more characteristic of suicide than of DSH; specific indicators of high risk include leaving a suicide note, continued determination to die, marked feelings of hopelessness, clear evidence of psychiatric illness (particularly severe depression), and an attempt carefully prepared with precautions against discovery and/or high lethality risk, either objectively or as imagined by the patient. In addition, risk is higher in older, male, unemployed or socially isolated subjects. Risk of repeated non-fatal DSH is highest in subjects of low social class, with antisocial personality disorder, no work and/or a criminal record, and in substance abusers.

Options for management
The objectives of DSH management are to decrease short-term risk of repetition and of completed suicide, to initiate or continue treatment of any underlying psychiatric illness (NB consider safety in overdose when prescribing antidepressants) and to address ongoing social difficulties. A good first step is to agree with the patient what their problems are, and what immediate interventions are both feasible and acceptable to them. Such a 'contract' can include a promise not to repeat any DSH. Only a small minority (usually where social support is lacking) need in-patient admission, although where suicide risk is high, compulsory admission may be indicated. Out-patient supportive psychotherapy (e.g. 'problem solving') may be helpful, as may referral to social services and/or voluntary agencies such as the Samaritans. In patients with affective disorder, lithium has been shown to reduce risk of both DSH and completed suicide. The frequency of repetitive DSH in the context of personality disorder may be reduced by depot neuroleptics.

Outcome
About 20% of self-harmers repeat their act within 1 year. Risk of actual suicide within 1 year is 1–2%, a 100-fold increase compared with the general population.

8 Stress reactions (including bereavement)

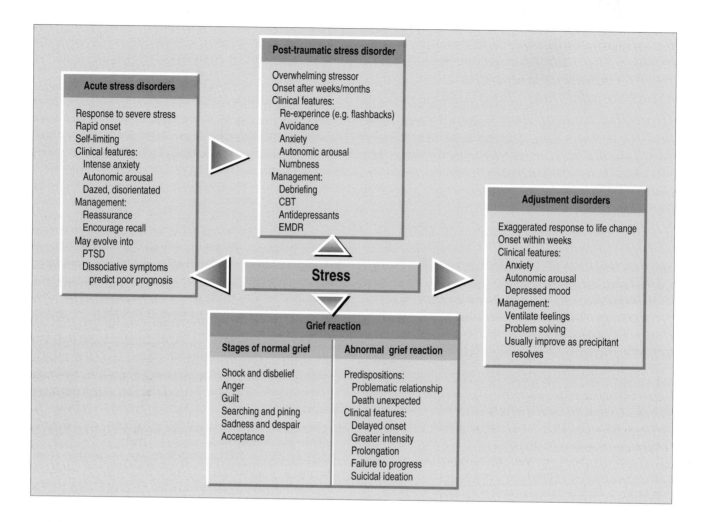

Major psychological stress involves threat or loss. Reactions to a broad range of major stressors (physical or sexual assault, transport accidents, natural disasters, war) are often similar in nature and involve emotional responses (fear from threat and sadness at loss), physical symptoms (autonomic arousal and/or fatigue), and psychological responses which may be conscious (e.g. avoidance behaviour) or unconscious (e.g. denial or dissociation). Abnormal stress reactions represent exaggerated or maladaptive responses. They may be acute and self-limiting or more prolonged (post-traumatic stress disorder (PTSD), adjustment disorder or abnormal grief).

Acute stress disorders (ASDs)

Acute stress disorders (ASDs) are rapid onset responses (within minutes or hours) to sudden and severe stressful events. Intense subjective anxiety is accompanied by autonomic arousal (sweating, dry mouth, tachycardia, vomiting). Survivors often feel dazed and perplexed, may be disorientated and can wander aimlessly. Purposeless overactivity, reduced sleep and nightmares are also common. Management involves reassurance and gentle encouragement to recall the traumatic events. Practical support may be required in dealing with underlying difficulties (e.g. temporary rehousing after a natural disaster). Anxiolytics (for a few days only) may give symptomatic relief. Dissociative symptoms carry a poor prognosis. Persistence of symptoms suggests the development of PTSD (see below).

Adjustment disorders

Adjustment disorders represent abnormal psychological responses to life changes such as job loss, house move or divorce. The onset is usually within weeks of the stressful event, but less severe than PTSD. Symptoms are similar, however, with a mixture of symptoms of anxiety (autonomic arousal, insomnia and irritability) and depression (sadness, tearfulness, worry). Biological features of depression are usually absent; indeed, the diagnosis should only be made where there are insufficient symptoms to justify a diagnosis of an anxiety or depressive disorder. Adjustment disorders usually improve following resolution of their precipitating cause.

Management involves encouragement to ventilate feelings and to develop appropriate coping mechanisms. Such help may focus on 'problem solving' in which patients are encouraged to form strategies to deal with particular problems.

Adjustment to chronic or terminal illness may manifest as anxiety, depression or exaggerated disability. There may be a sequence (similar to that in bereavement as described below) of shock and denial (and search for an ever-elusive 'cure'), followed by anger, sadness and finally acceptance. Principles of management involve adequate symptomatic (particularly pain) control, honest explanation (which may have to be offered repeatedly until the patient is emotionally ready to understand it), supportive psychotherapy and family counselling.

PTSD

The onset of PTSD may occur weeks, months or (rarely) years after the stressful experience (the nature of which may, as in ASD, include assault, accident, disaster or battle). DSM-IV and ICD-10 require that the stressor be exceptionally severe for PTSD to be diagnosed, but the pattern of symptoms and signs may be similar in subjects experiencing more minor stress. A duration of symptoms for one month is required to make the diagnosis. The characteristic features of PTSD involve

1 *Persistent intrusive thinking or re-experiencing* of the trauma, such as waking 'flashbacks' or nightmares.
2 *Avoidance* of reminders of the event (e.g. accident victims not going near the scene of the accident).
3 Persistent *anxiety* with autonomic symptoms, hypervigilance, sleep disturbance, irritability and poor concentration.
4 *Numbness* (loss of interest in everyday activities or even in loving relationships).

There is considerable symptomatic overlap between PTSD and depression (see Chapter 5); the latter may also be precipitated by extreme stress and may coexist with PTSD.

Risk of developing PTSD is proportional to the magnitude of the stressor, but may be greater following 'man-made' rather than natural disasters and if some degree of stress continues. People with pre-existing psychiatric illness or personality difficulties appear more vulnerable to developing PTSD.

Symptoms of PTSD may persist for the rest of the victim's life—as occurred in many Holocaust survivors. Antidepressant drugs (even in the absence of major depressive disorder), cognitive behavioural therapy (CBT) and the specific technique of Eye Movement Desensitization and Reprocessing (EMDR) have been shown in controlled clinical trials to be effective. The widely used technique of debriefing (in which patients are encouraged to recall the stressful events in detail and supported through the associated emotions) immediately after the trauma was thought to prevent subsequent PTSD, but is probably ineffective.

Bereavement and grief

The loss of a spouse or close relative is the most universally experienced extreme stress. Bereavement is associated with increased mortality (from cardiovascular disease and cancer) and may precipitate depression and even suicide.

'Normal' grief often follows a recognizable sequence of stages that last for up to 2 years. The initial reaction to bereavement (lasting days or a few weeks) is of *shock and disbelief* with autonomic arousal but usually without psychological fear. There may be paroxysms of weeping. This may be followed by feelings of *anger* at being deserted by the deceased relative, and *guilt and self-blame* for not having done more for them. The next stage consists of *'searching' or 'pining'*, vivid dreams that the dead person is still alive and, often, pseudo-hallucinations (usually at night) of the dead person speaking to them. *Sadness and despair* follow this, accompanied by many of the features (poor sleep and appetite, social withdrawal) of depression. Finally, there is *acceptance* that the deceased will not come back and a regaining of interests. Symptoms often recur briefly on anniversaries.

'Abnormal' grief is characterized by delayed onset of grief, greater intensity of symptoms, or prolongation of the reaction, subjects often getting 'stuck' at one of the stages of grieving. Suicidal ideas may be harboured during abnormal pining (a wish to be with the deceased again) or despair. Abnormal grief is more likely where the relationship with the deceased was problematic (ambivalent or overinvolved), where the death was sudden and where normal grieving is impeded by social constraints such as 'having to put on a brave face for the children'.

Normal grieving requires no specific management apart from support and encouragement to ventilate feelings and accept them as normal. Abnormal grief reactions may respond to a cognitive–behavioural approach, encouraging structured review of the relationship and giving vent to the emotions produced. Antidepressants may be indicated if depressive symptoms are prominent and persistent; significant suicidal ideation may warrant hospitalization.

9 Anxiety disorders

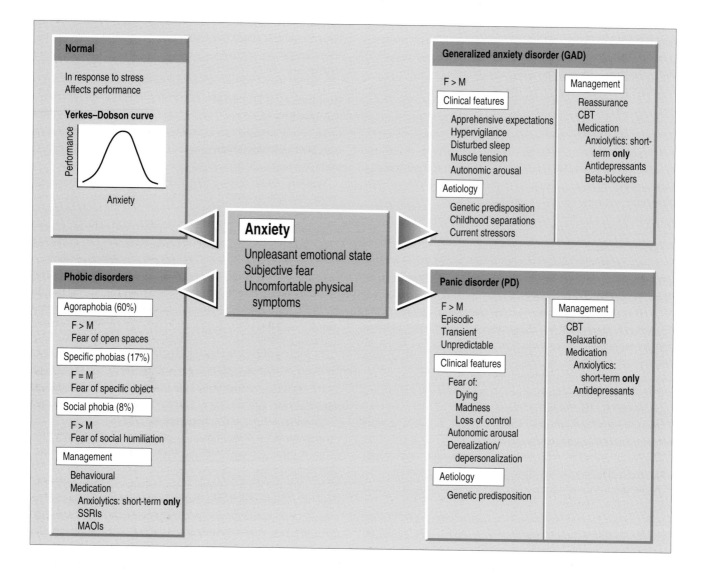

Normal

In response to stress
Affects performance

Yerkes–Dobson curve

Performance / Anxiety

Phobic disorders

Agoraphobia (60%)

F > M
Fear of open spaces

Specific phobias (17%)

F = M
Fear of specific object

Social phobia (8%)

F > M
Fear of social humiliation

Management

Behavioural
Medication
  Anxiolytics: short-term **only**
  SSRIs
  MAOIs

Anxiety

Unpleasant emotional state
Subjective fear
Uncomfortable physical symptoms

Generalized anxiety disorder (GAD)

F > M

Clinical features

Apprehensive expectations
Hypervigilance
Disturbed sleep
Muscle tension
Autonomic arousal

Aetiology

Genetic predisposition
Childhood separations
Current stressors

Management

Reassurance
CBT
Medication
  Anxiolytics: short-term **only**
  Antidepressants
  Beta-blockers

Panic disorder (PD)

F > M
Episodic
Transient
Unpredictable

Clinical features

Fear of:
  Dying
  Madness
  Loss of control
Autonomic arousal
Derealization/
  depersonalization

Aetiology

Genetic predisposition

Management

CBT
Relaxation
Medication
  Anxiolytics:
    short-term **only**
  Antidepressants

Definition and classification

Anxiety is an unpleasant emotional state accompanied by a subjective experience of fear, bodily discomfort and physical symptoms which may be accompanied by a feeling of impending threat or death in the future, and which may or may not be in response to a recognizable threat. Anxiety is usually a normal phenomenon which occurs in response to stress and, with optimum levels, can be beneficial (Yerkes–Dobson curve; no anxiety = no performance; increasing anxiety = increasing performance; too much anxiety = deterioration in performance). Pathological anxiety can present in discrete attacks with no external stimulus (panic disorder), in discrete attacks with stimuli (phobias) or in a generalized, persistent state (generalized anxiety disorder (GAD)). Anxiety can, however, also occur as part of other disorders (e.g. depression).

Panic disorder

Panic disorder is characterized by recurrent episodic severe panic (anxiety) attacks (PA) which occur unpredictably and are not restricted to any particular situation or set of circumstances (although certain situations such as being in crowds may become associated with them). The dominant symptoms, varying from individual to individual, include discrete periods of intense fear, impending doom or discomfort, accompanied by palpitations, tachycardia, a pounding heart, sweating, trembling, dyspnoea, feeling of choking, chest pain/discomfort, nausea/abdominal discomfort, dizziness, derealization (the experience of the world or people in it seeming lifeless), depersonalization (being detached from oneself), fear of losing control, 'going crazy' or dying, paraesthesias, chills and hot flushes. Typically, the duration of a PA is only a few minutes. A complication is the development of 'anticipatory fear' of helplessness (or loss of control) during an attack, with the result that the individual may be reluctant to be alone in a public place or away from home. Both current classificatory systems (DSM-IV; ICD-10) stipulate at least three PAs in a 3-week period where there is no discernable objective danger to the individual, who must be free of anxiety between the discrete PAs. Of the population, 0.8% have panic disorder; women are affected more than men and the typical age at onset is 25–44 years. Panic disorder shows familial transmission which breeds true (i.e. is unrelated to GAD). Sodium lactate infusion and breathing carbon dioxide induce PA in susceptible individuals. Treatment includes exposure and CBT (see Chapter 32), breathing exercises, benzodiazepines (NB tolerance, addiction), antidepressants (imipramine, phenelzine, SSRIs).

Generalized anxiety disorder

This is characterized by generalized, persistent, excessive anxiety or worry (apprehensive expectation) about a number of events (e.g. work, school performance) which the individual finds difficult to control, lasting for more than 6 months. The anxiety is usually associated with subjective apprehension (fears, worries), increased vigilance, feeling restless and on edge, sleeping difficulties (initial/middle insomnia, fatigue on waking), motor tension (tremor, hyperactive deep reflexes) and autonomic hyperactivity (tachycardia, tachypnoea, dilated pupils). GAD may be acute (sudden onset, occurring as a reaction to severe external stress and, in relatively stable personalities, short course, good prognosis, resolving completely) or chronic (prolonged course, waxing/waning, may or may not be a reaction to stressful external events). The symptoms are essentially the same in the two types. The prognosis is worse for chronic GAD; males and individuals with premorbid stability do better. Complications include secondary agoraphobia, depression, alcohol and drug abuse. GAD occurs in 2–4% of the general population, in 27% of psychiatric consultations in general practice and in 8% of psychiatric out-patients. It usually begins in early adult life, and affects women more than men. Aetiological factors include a genetic predisposition, childhood experiences characterized by separations, demands for high achievement and excess conformity, current stressful life events and biological factors (dysfunction of autonomic nervous system reflecting increased sympathetic tone or parasympathetic abnormalities). Several psychophysiological measures are increased in GAD including pulse, skin conduction, forearm blood flow and muscular tension (measured by an electromyogram (EMG)). On the EEG, the alpha rhythm is decreased. Psychological treatments include reassurance, counselling and psychotherapy. Specific psychotherapeutic approaches include CBT (identify morbid anticipatory thoughts and replace with realistic cognitions), insight orientated therapy (explore conflicts) and anxiety management (distraction techniques, breathing and relaxation exercises). Medications include short-term judicious use of benzodiazepines (NB tolerance, addiction), tricyclic antidepressants (which are not addictive, e.g. imipramine) and beta-blockers (e.g. propanolol). In a few resistant cases, psychosurgery may help. Differential diagnosis includes thyrotoxicosis, parathyroid disease, phaeochromocytoma, carcinoid syndrome, hypoglycaemia, withdrawal from drugs and/ or alcohol, depression, schizophrenia and excessive caffeine ingestion.

Phobic disorders

Phobic disorders are divided into specific or simple phobias, social phobia and agoraphobia. In these, fear is out of proportion to the situation, cannot be reasoned or explained away, is beyond voluntary control, is recognized by the individual as being excessive and results in avoidance of the feared situations.

Agoraphobia (also known as phobic anxiety/depersonalization), accounts for 60% of phobic patients seen by psychiatrists (66% female, age at onset 15–35 years) and is characterized by anxiety about being in places or situations from which escape might be difficult or in which help may not be available in the event of having a situationally predisposed PA (e.g. being outside home alone, in a crowd, out shopping, on a bridge, in a bus, train or car). The PA-inducing situations are avoided or the presence of a companion is secured.

Specific phobias (17% of phobic patients seen by psychiatrists; female and male prevalence equal) include fear induced by the presence or anticipation of a specific object or situation (e.g. flying, heights, animals, seeing blood).

Social phobia (8% of phobic patients seen by psychiatrists; 60% women; onset usually after puberty) results in a marked persistent fear of social performance situations in which the individual is exposed to unfamiliar people or to possible scrutiny by others and fears that he/she will act in a way that will be humiliating or embarrassing (e.g. blushing, shaking, vomiting). It is probably not a homogeneous clinical entity. Treatment includes behavioural techniques (exposure by systematic desensitization, flooding, or modelling), medication (e.g. short-term benzodiazepines, beta-blockers, SSRIs, phenelzine) and psychotherapy which may be supportive (to ensure readjustment of lifestyle) or psychodynamic (exploring conflicts, secondary gain, family approaches).

Mitral valve prolapse (MVP)

Investigations have suggested an increased incidence (40–50%) of MVP in people with panic disorder or agoraphobia (prevalence in general population = 6–20%). MVP does not cause PA (if panic disorder is treated successfully, MVP persists). MVP and panic disorder may both form part of a syndrome of primary autonomic dysfunction, or MVP may act as an autonomic precipitant in individuals with a genetic predisposition to panic disorder.

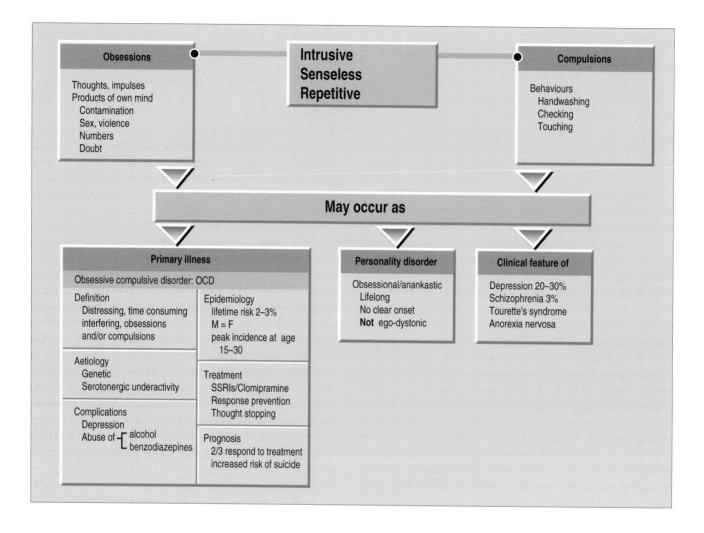

Definition

Obsessions are unwelcome, persistent, recurrent ideas, thoughts, impulses or images which are intrusive, senseless and uncomfortable (egodystonic) for the individual, who attempts to suppress or neutralize them and recognizes them as absurd and a product of his/her own mind. Common obsessions include unpleasant thoughts of blasphemy, sex, violence, contamination, numbers and doubt. Obsessions may take the form of thoughts, images (vivid, morbid or violent scenes), ruminations (continuous pondering), doubts and obsessional slowness. Rarer obsessions include arithmomania (counting), onomatomania (the desire to utter a forbidden word) and *folie de pourquoi* (the irresistible habit of seeking explanations for commonplace facts by asking perpetual questions). Obsessions should be distinguished from impulses (thoughts which are not displeasurable (egosyntonic)) and rituals (actions which have a magical quality and are culturally sanctioned).

Compulsions are repetitive, purposeful behaviours performed with reluctance in response to an obsession, according to certain rules in a stereotyped fashion, and designed to neutralize or prevent discomfort or a dreaded event. The activity is excessive and not connected to the thought (obsession) in a realistic way. The individual realizes that this egodystonic behaviour is unreasonable. Common compulsions include handwashing, cleaning, counting, checking, touching and constant rearrangement of objects to achieve symmetry.

If resistance to the obsessions or compulsions is attempted, anxiety usually increases until the compulsive activity is performed.

Mild obsessions and compulsions are common in the general population. More severe obsessions and compulsions are prominent symptoms in primary OCD, they also occur in the obsessional (anankastic) personality disorder, are common in depression, schizophrenia and Tourette's syndrome (TS) and may occur in puerperal illness (fear of harming baby), anorexia nervosa, Generalised Anxiety Disorder, dementia, temporal lobe epilepsy, Parkinson's disease, Sydenham's chorea (chorea associated with rheumatic fever), head injury and manganese poisoning.

Anankastic personality disorder

Characteristic features include rigidity of thinking, perfectionism, orderliness, moralistic preoccupation with rules, excessive cleanliness and a tendency to hoard. These are egosyntonic life traits with no obvious onset. The perfectionism may interfere with the affected subjects' ability to complete tasks and objectively high standards are seldom achieved. Subjects are often emotionally cold.

Obsessive-compulsive disorder

Classification

OCD is currently classified under the anxiety disorders, but there is increasing evidence suggesting that this is inappropriate, as the disorders have different sex ratios, ages at onset and responses to medication (e.g. benzodiazepines, tricyclic antidepressants).

Clinical characteristics

OCD is characterized by egodystonic, time-consuming (take up >1 hour/day) obsessions and compulsions which interfere with the individual's everyday functioning. Avoidance of stimuli or activities that trigger obsessive–compulsive symptoms is very common. Resistance is characteristic but may not persist. Onset is usually during adolescence. The commonest obsessions are concerned with contamination (43%); handwashing is the commonest compulsion (85%). A premorbid obsessional personality is present in 70% of cases. Complications include depression and abuse of anxiolytics or alcohol. Severe OCD can lead to as much distress and functional impairment as any psychotic illness.

Epidemiology

The Epidemiological Catchment Area (ECA) studies suggest a lifetime prevalence of 1.9–3.2%. Males and females are affected equally.

Aetiology

Causal theories of OCD have changed considerably in the last 30 years. Psychoanalytic theory postulated it to represent a defence against cruel and aggressive fantasies: filling the mind with obsessional thoughts prevents undesirable ideas from entering consciousness. It was also thought to be a defensive regression to a pregenital anal–erotic stage of development. Behaviourists proposed that compulsive behaviour was learned and maintained by operant conditioning processes, the anxiety reduction following the compulsive behaviour strengthening

it. More recently, biological factors have been emphasized. In many patients there are genetic influences with a positive family history of OCD (in 50% of cases), tics or TS. It is thought that there are three types of OCD: (i) genetic and breeding true; (ii) genetic and related to tics or TS; (iii) non-familial form. Biochemical abnormalities (especially involving serotonin) are now thought to be important in the pathophysiology of OCD. Brain neuroimaging techniques have shown functional abnormalities in frontal cortex and basal ganglia.

Management

Traditionally, CBT has been the mainstay of treatment of OCD, but pharmacological therapy has become increasingly important. CBT includes exposure followed by response prevention for compulsions, and both habituation training and thought-stopping for obsessions. During exposure and response prevention, the patient is instructed to desist from performing the unwanted compulsive behaviour (e.g. repeated handwashing) while simultaneously being exposed to a situation (e.g. wiping a lavatory seat) likely to increase the need to perform it. Habituation training involves repeated exposure to obsessional thoughts (e.g. the patient listens to a cassette tape continuously repeating out loud his/her obsessional thoughts) without allowing them to be neutralized until the individual habituates and the anxiety decreases. The opposite to habituation training is thought stopping (well known but less effective), during which the patient is encouraged to relax and ruminate until the obsessions are uppermost in his/her mind. The therapist then shouts 'Stop!' and the patient tries to stop ruminating. The procedure can be enhanced by a mildly aversive or painful stimulus (such as the patient pulling on a rubber band round his/her wrist) experienced at the same time as the command. Eventually, the patient learns to stop the thoughts autonomously. Drug treatment (which may be most effective in conjunction with CBT) is with antidepressants which act specifically on serotonin, such as clomipramine and the SSRIs. These drugs are effective even in the absence of coexistent depressive symptomatology. Overall response to CBT and/or drugs is about 60%; in contrast, placebo responses in clinical trials are very low (5%). The augmentation of an SSRI by antipsychotics may be useful in the treatment of both obsessions and compulsions. Psychosurgery (cingulotomy) is rarely used but may be effective in the most severe and treatment-resistant cases.

Course and prognosis

OCD is chronic with waxing and waning of symptoms. Patients with compulsions only and those with severe symptoms, persistent life stresses or premorbid obsessional personality fare worst. Traditionally, OCD was thought to carry a low risk of suicide; recently, however, the suicide rate (particularly in subjects with coexistent depressive illness) has been found to be considerable.

11 Eating disorders

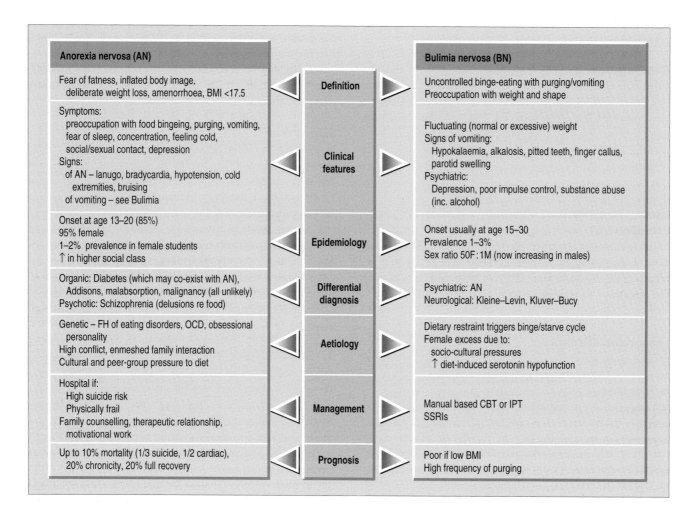

Anorexia nervosa (AN)		Bulimia nervosa (BN)
Fear of fatness, inflated body image, deliberate weight loss, amenorrhoea, BMI <17.5	**Definition**	Uncontrolled binge-eating with purging/vomiting Preoccupation with weight and shape
Symptoms: preoccupation with food bingeing, purging, vomiting, fear of sleep, concentration, feeling cold, social/sexual contact, depression Signs: of AN – lanugo, bradycardia, hypotension, cold extremities, bruising of vomiting – see Bulimia	**Clinical features**	Fluctuating (normal or excessive) weight Signs of vomiting: Hypokalaemia, alkalosis, pitted teeth, finger callus, parotid swelling Psychiatric: Depression, poor impulse control, substance abuse (inc. alcohol)
Onset at age 13–20 (85%) 95% female 1–2% prevalence in female students ↑ in higher social class	**Epidemiology**	Onset usually at age 15–30 Prevalence 1–3% Sex ratio 50F : 1M (now increasing in males)
Organic: Diabetes (which may co-exist with AN), Addisons, malabsorption, malignancy (all unlikely) Psychotic: Schizophrenia (delusions re food)	**Differential diagnosis**	Psychiatric: AN Neurological: Kleine–Levin, Kluver–Bucy
Genetic – FH of eating disorders, OCD, obsessional personality High conflict, enmeshed family interaction Cultural and peer-group pressure to diet	**Aetiology**	Dietary restraint triggers binge/starve cycle Female excess due to: socio-cultural pressures ↑ diet-induced serotonin hypofunction
Hospital if: High suicide risk Physically frail Family counselling, therapeutic relationship, motivational work	**Management**	Manual based CBT or IPT SSRIs
Up to 10% mortality (1/3 suicide, 1/2 cardiac), 20% chronicity, 20% full recovery	**Prognosis**	Poor if low BMI High frequency of purging

Anorexia nervosa (AN)

AN is characterized by a morbid fear of fatness, deliberate weight loss, distorted body image, amenorrhoea and a Body Mass Index (BMI—defined as weight (kg)/ht (m)^2) of less than 17.5.

Associated clinical features include preoccupation with food (dieting, often with specific carbohydrate avoidance, and sometimes preparation of elaborate meals for others), hyperactivity (with vigorous exercise to lose weight), constipation, cold intolerance, social isolation, body disparagement, fear of sexuality, depressive symptoms and obsessive–compulsive (often perfectionistic) phenomena. Self-consciousness about eating in public and more generalized social isolation are often found. Sufferers usually fall into 'restrictive' (minimal food intake and exercise) or 'bulimic' (episodic binge eating with laxative use and induced vomiting) subtypes. Extreme emaciation is often disguised by make-up and baggy clothes. On examination, the skin is usually dry and yellow and the trunk and face

may be covered in fine 'lanugo' hair. Bradycardia, hypotension, anaemia and osteoporosis are common. Leucopenia is frequently found. Consequences of repeated vomiting include hypokalaemia, alkalosis, pitted teeth, parotid swelling and scarring of the dorsum of the hand.

There is a preponderance in women of 95%; 85% have an onset at age 13–20 years. AN is increasingly being seen in children, where the sex ratio is nearly equal. AN in men has a somewhat later onset (typically 17–24 years). Overall prevalence rates of about 1–2% in schoolgirls and female university students have been reported. Higher rates are found in higher socio-economic classes; this may reflect differences in access to services.

Aetiological factors include precipitation by puberty and by stress. A genetic component is indicated by the higher concordance for AN in monozygotic (60%) than dizygotic (10%) twins, as well as by the high positive family history of eating disorders, obsessive–compulsive disorders and obsessional personality. Desire to avoid the consequences of sexual maturity has been implicated. Family difficulties (particularly an enmeshed pattern of family interaction and poor conflict resolution) are effects rather causes of the AN.

Differential diagnosis includes organic causes of low weight (e.g. diabetes mellitus, Addison's disease, malabsorption). These conditions are not usually associated with abnormal attitudes to weight or eating. Diabetes may coexist with AN. Psychiatric causes of low weight include depression (which may also coexist with AN), and psychotic disorders (including schizophrenia) in which there may be delusions concerning food, substance and alcohol abuse. There is an important overlap between AN and bulimia nervosa (see below).

Management initially involves exclusion of other diagnoses and identification of treatable coexistent depression. The development of therapeutic relationship and motivational counselling are important elements in AN management. Hospitalization (sometimes compulsory) may be necessary if weight loss has been rapid, if there is significant suicide risk or if there is significant cardiac or cognitive failure. A target weight and weight-gain schedule may initially involve bed rest with supervised high-calorie feeding. Patients frequently sabotage such programmes by discarding food and/or purging and vomiting secretly. A behavioural reward programme for successful weight gain is sometimes used. Drugs which speed gastric emptying (metoclopramide, cisapride) may reduce bloating and facilitate refeeding. Fluoxetine may be helpful in maintaining weight gain.

Prognosis is variable. Short-term response to treatment is usually good but about 20% fail to recover. Mortality may be as high as 10% (1/2 cardiac; 1/3 suicide). About 20% recover completely and the remainder have a chronic fluctuating course, frequently developing bulimia.

Bulimia nervosa (BN)

The core feature of BN is binge eating (which may be as much as 20 000 kCal in a session) with an associated sense of loss of control, and compensatory vomiting and/or purging. Fasting, laxatives and diuretics are also often used. Milder Binge Eating Disorder (BED) may occur at a normal or high BMI. Preoccupation with body weight and shape is also crucial as in AN.

Associated clinical features include normal or excessive weight (often with major fluctuations), and the stigmata of excessive vomiting. Sufferers may describe a trance-like state during bingeing. Amenorrhoea occurs in 50% (despite normal weight). As in AN, strict dieting and exercise are often resorted to for weight control. Hypokalaemia may lead to dysrhythmias or to renal damage; acute oesophageal tears can occur during forced vomiting. Psychiatric features include intense self-loathing (especially after an episode of bingeing) and associated depression; substance abuse and poor impulse control are also associated.

Binge eating is very common in adolescence; the prevalence of true BN is 1–3%, with a 50 : 1 female preponderance. Presentation is somewhat later than for AN (usually in the late teens or twenties), although onset is often in the mid-teens.

Aetiological features include dietary restraint (to which women are more socio-culturally prone) triggering a binge–starve cycle which may in turn reduce serotonergic tone (more markedly in women). There is an excess of alcohol and substance abuse and depression, as well as of BN itself, in first-degree relatives of subjects with BN.

Differential diagnosis must consider AN and affective disorder (including cyclothymia) as well as obesity. Specific (rare) neurological causes of overeating include Kleine–Levin (associated hypersomnia) and Kluver–Bucy (compulsive orality and hypersexuality) syndromes. Diabetic women with BN may use their diabetes to lose weight.

Management involves medical stabilization and psychotherapy (usually CBT or IPT; see Chapter 32) to establish a regular eating programme, re-establish control of diet and address underlying negative cognitions. Antidepressants have an independent anti-bulimic effect, best established for fluoxetine (60 mg).

Prognosis is poor in patients with low BMI and with a high frequency of purging. The short-term benefits of treatment are, however, reasonably well established, with CBT or IPT giving about 50% remission.

Obesity

This is defined as a BMI >30. Its prevalence is culturally variable (very high in USA). Mild to moderate (but not severe) obesity is commoner in females and with increasing age. The main aetiological factors are family and cultural norms, though there is increasing recent interest in weight-controlling genes (egleptins, obgenes). Management involves a behavioural and educational programme to reestablish sensible eating, and cognitive and/or supportive psychotherapy addressing secondary low self-esteem that may otherwise perpetuate the overeating. Appetite suppressants (e.g. fenfluramine) are only of short-term benefit. Surgical treatment (jaw wiring, gastric resection or bypass) is indicated in severe refractory cases. It is increasingly recognized that BED without severe restraint or vomiting may lead to obesity; patients require similar treatment to BN.

Pica

Pica is defined as the persistent eating of non-nutritive substances (such as coal or soil). It is normal in very young children and mild forms are often seen in pregnancy. Its persistence may reflect underlying nutritional deficiency or psychiatric illness—particularly learning disability, autism or schizophrenia. Management involves treatment of any underlying condition and a behavioural modification programme.

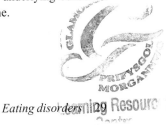

12 Disorders of personality

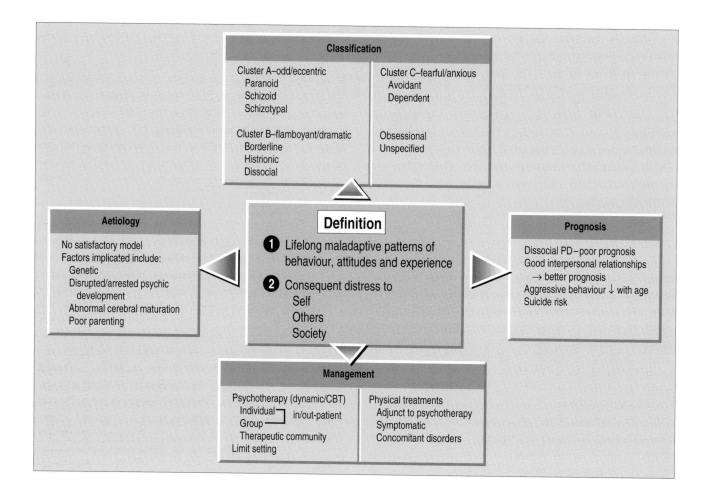

Classification

Cluster A–odd/eccentric
Paranoid
Schizoid
Schizotypal

Cluster B–flamboyant/dramatic
Borderline
Histrionic
Dissocial

Cluster C–fearful/anxious
Avoidant
Dependent

Obsessional
Unspecified

Aetiology

No satisfactory model
Factors implicated include:
Genetic
Disrupted/arrested psychic
development
Abnormal cerebral maturation
Poor parenting

Definition

1 Lifelong maladaptive patterns of
behaviour, attitudes and experience

2 Consequent distress to
Self
Others
Society

Prognosis

Dissocial PD–poor prognosis
Good interpersonal relationships
→ better prognosis
Aggressive behaviour ↓ with age
Suicide risk

Management

Psychotherapy (dynamic/CBT)
Individual ┐ in/out-patient
Group ┘
Therapeutic community
Limit setting

Physical treatments
Adjunct to psychotherapy
Symptomatic
Concomitant disorders

Definition

Both ICD-10 and DSM-IV define personality disorders (PDs) as persistent, lifelong, deeply ingrained maladaptive patterns of inner experience and behaviour which are the expression of an individual's lifestyle and deviate markedly from the expectations of his/her culture. PDs usually arise early in the individual's development and persist into adulthood. They are frequently associated with subjective/personal distress and/or have adverse effects on interpersonal relations and/or society. PDs are characterized by problems in cognition (ways of perceiving and interpreting self, others, events), affectivity (range, intensity, appropriateness of affective response), interpersonal functioning, impulse control, and occupational and social performance.

Assessment of personality

Personality assessments include self report measures such as the Personality Diagnostic Questionnaire (PDQ) and structured interviews (e.g. Structured Clinical Interview for Personality Disorders (SCID); Personality Assessment Schedule (PAS)).

Epidemiology

Ten per cent of the adult population have a PD of at least mild severity as do 20% of general practitioner (GP) attenders, 30% of psychiatric out-patients and 40% of psychiatric in-patients. PD is consistently more common in subjects of low social class. Prevalence of some sub-categories decrease with age.

Aetiology

There is no satisfactory aetiological model for PD. Factors implicated include genetic influences (monozygotic/dizygotic concordance; XYY individuals display increased criminality irrespective of IQ or socio-economic class). Psychodynamic theories suggest that PDs result from disrupted/arrested psychic development (e.g. defective and infantile ego functions; defective object relations). Adverse intrauterine, perinatal or postnatal factors leading to abnormal cerebral maturation may predispose to PD, as may poor parenting and social reinforcement of abnormal behaviours. An underactive autonomic nervous system has been implicated in dissocial PD.

Classification and characteristics

The clinical characteristics of specific PDs, grouped (following DSM-IV) into three clusters, are summarized below. It should be noted that patients (particularly those with severe PD) may fulfil criteria for more than one PD diagnosis.

Cluster 'A' (odd/eccentric)

1 Paranoid PD: cold affect, pervasive distrust, suspiciousness of others, preoccupation with doubts about the fidelity or trustworthiness of friends/spouse, reluctance to confide, bearing grudges, reading negative meanings into remarks, hypersensitivity to rebuffs and a grandiose sense of personal rights.

2 Schizoid PD: social withdrawal, a restricted range of emotional expression, little interest in sex, restricted pleasure, lacking confidantes, indifference to praise or criticism, aloofness and insensitivity to social norms.

3 Schizotypal PD: pervasive social and interpersonal deficits, ideas of reference, magical thinking, unusual perceptions (e.g. bodily illusions), vague, circumstantial, tangential thinking, suspiciousness, inappropriate/constricted affect, eccentricity and excessive social anxiety. Schizotypal PDs are more common in relatives of people with schizophrenia.

Cluster 'B' (flamboyant/dramatic)

1 Borderline PD (impulsive): unstable and intense interpersonal relationships, self-image and affect, self-damaging impulsivity (spending, sex, substance abuse, reckless driving, binge eating), identity confusion, chronic anhedonia, recurrent suicidal or self-mutilating behaviour, transient paranoid ideation and frantic efforts to avoid real or imagined abandonment.

2 Histrionic PD (narcissistic): excessive shallow emotionality, attention seeking, suggestibility, shallow/labile affect, inappropriate sexual seductiveness but frigidity and immaturity, narcissism, grandiosity, exploitative actions.

3 Dissocial PD (antisocial; psychopathic; sociopathic): persistent disregard for the rights or safety of others, gross irresponsibility, incapacity for maintaining relationships, irritability, low frustration tolerance and aggressive threshold, incapacity to experience guilt or profit from experience, deceitfulness, impulsivity, disregard for personal safety, proneness to blame others. Dissocial PD is important legally; in some countries (e.g. UK) it can justify detention under the Mental Health Act (MHA; see Chapter 29).

Cluster 'C' (fearful/anxious)

1 Avoidant PD (anxious): persistent feelings of tension and inadequacy, social inhibition, unwillingness to become involved with people unless certain of being liked and restriction in lifestyle to maintain physical security.

2 Dependent PD (asthenic): an excessive need to be taken care of leading to submissive and clinging behaviour, fears of separation, difficulty in making everyday decisions without excessive advice, needing others to assume responsibility, difficulty in expressing disagreement for fear of loss of support/approval, difficulty in initiating projects (because of lack of self-confidence), going to lengths to gain support from others, constantly needing close relationships, undue compliance with other's wishes, unwilling to make demands on people and preoccupation with fears of being left alone.

Other PDs include **obsessional** (anankastic; see Chapter 10) and **unspecified**.

Management

Successful management depends on securing an adequate treatment alliance so that the patient is able to work together with a therapist. Deep-seated mistrust and ambivalence therefore need to be addressed early in treatment, and the long-term and arduous nature of treatment should be discussed with the patient at the outset. Multidisciplinary and multiagency work is often required. Admission to hospital during periods of crisis may be necessary.

Specific therapeutic techniques include interpretative psychotherapy (individual, group, therapeutic community; see Chapter 32), and CBT. Limit-setting and confrontation are important adjuncts. Physical treatments have not been adequately evaluated but are useful in treating coexisting conditions (e.g. depression) and in the management of acute subjective distress, particularly in an out-patient setting where underlying conflicts cannot immediately be addressed. Drug treatment is usually symptom focused. Antipsychotics may be useful for cognitive symptoms (e.g. ideas of reference, depersonalization) impulsivity and intense angry affect. They may also alleviate the abnormal mood (empty, lonely, bored) associated with some PDs. Monoamine oxidase inhibitors (MAOIs) may be helpful in some borderline PDs, particularly where there is a history of childhood hyperactivity. Carbamazepine and lithium may help some individuals with episodic behavioural dyscontrol and aggression, even in the absence of epileptic, affective or organic features. Drug treatment and psychotherapy in PD are not mutually exclusive.

In the UK, the MHA allows detention of individuals with PDs who are dangerous and violent (e.g. who have committed crimes) in special hospitals or therapeutic prisons.

Prognosis

In general, individuals with PDs show decreased aggressive behaviour with age, although the ability to form successful interpersonal relationships remains poor. Borderline PD carries a relatively favourable prognosis, with clinical recovery in over 50% at 10–25-year follow-up; schizoid and schizotypal patients tend to remain isolated. Dissocial PD carries a particularly poor prognosis. Certain individuals with PDs may relieve subjective discomfort by abusing alcohol and psychoactive substances, resulting in dependence. There is an increased risk of suicide in people with PDs; between 30 and 60% of completed suicides have evidence of PD.

Obsessional PDs are at high risk of progression to OCD (see Chapter 10) or to depression; paranoid and schizotypal PD may progress to schizophrenia. In contrast, schizoid PD does not predispose to schizophrenia. Some PDs may confer susceptibility to physical illness (e.g. obsessional PD and duodenal ulcer).

13 Substance misuse

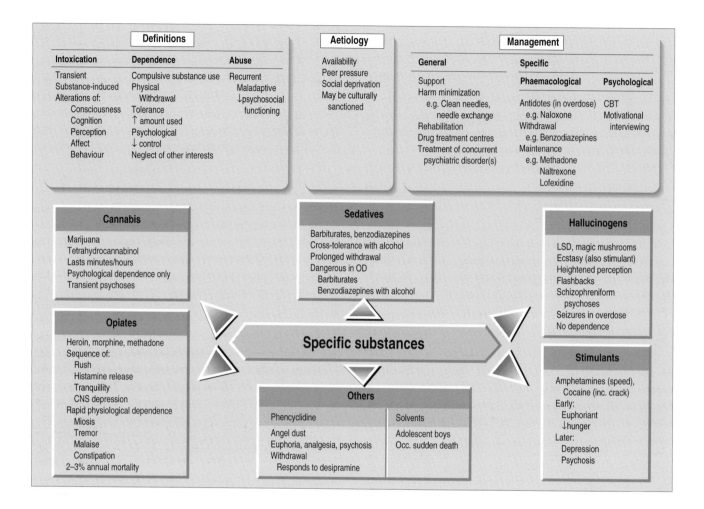

Definitions		
Intoxication	**Dependence**	**Abuse**
Transient	Compulsive substance use	Recurrent
Substance-induced	Physical	Maladaptive
Alterations of:	Withdrawal	↓psychosocial
Consciousness	Tolerance	functioning
Cognition	↑ amount used	
Perception	Psychological	
Affect	↓ control	
Behaviour	Neglect of other interests	

Aetiology

Availability
Peer pressure
Social deprivation
May be culturally
  sanctioned

Management		
General	**Specific**	
	Phaemacological	**Psychological**
Support		
Harm minimization	Antidotes (in overdose)	CBT
e.g. Clean needles,	e.g. Naloxone	Motivational
needle exchange	Withdrawal	interviewing
Rehabilitation	e.g. Benzodiazepines	
Drug treatment centres	Maintenance	
Treatment of concurrent	e.g. Methadone	
psychiatric disorder(s)	Naltrexone	
	Lofexidine	

Cannabis

Marijuana
Tetrahydrocannabinol
Lasts minutes/hours
Psychological dependence only
Transient psychoses

Opiates

Heroin, morphine, methadone
Sequence of:
  Rush
  Histamine release
  Tranquillity
  CNS depression
Rapid physiological dependence
  Miosis
  Tremor
  Malaise
  Constipation
2–3% annual mortality

Sedatives

Barbiturates, benzodiazepines
Cross-tolerance with alcohol
Prolonged withdrawal
Dangerous in OD
  Barbiturates
  Benzodiazepines with alcohol

Specific substances

Others

Phencyclidine	Solvents
Angel dust	Adolescent boys
Euphoria, analgesia, psychosis	Occ. sudden death
Withdrawal	
Responds to desipramine	

Hallucinogens

LSD, magic mushrooms
Ecstasy (also stimulant)
Heightened perception
Flashbacks
Schizophreniform
  psychoses
Seizures in overdose
No dependence

Stimulants

Amphetamines (speed),
  Cocaine (inc. crack)
Early:
  Euphoriant
  ↓hunger
Later:
  Depression
  Psychosis

Acute intoxication refers to transient disturbances of consciousness, cognition, perception, affect or behaviour following the administration of a psychoactive substance (PS). *Harmful* PS use implies damage to health.

Dependence involves physiological and/or psychological elements. The former include a withdrawal state, tolerance (increasing doses of PSs needed for the same effect), and the PS being taken in larger amounts or for longer than was intended. Psychological dependence involves a sense of compulsion to take the PS, difficulties in controlling PS use, increasing time spent obtaining, ingesting or recovering from the PS, persistence with PS use despite awareness of harmful consequences, a persistent but futile wish to cut down PS use and/or reduction in important social, occupational or recreational activities because of PS use.

Substance abuse (maladaptive and recurrent PS use leading to significant impairment or distress) may involve failure to fulfil obligations at work/school/home, hazardous behaviour (e.g. driving a car) and legal problems (e.g. arrests).

Aetiology and management

Socio-environmental factors (availability, peer pressure, deprivation) are the main determinants of PS use, but neurobiological mechanisms, pre-existing psychopathology (e.g. attention-deficit disorder rendering an individual vulnerable to cocaine use), PDs (borderline or antisocial), iatrogenic factors (e.g. prescribed benzodiazepines, (BDZs)), conditioned learning and the pharmacological properties of the PS may all contribute. The majority of PS misusers have disorders of personality and at least 20% have other psychiatric disorders (dual diagnosis (DD)). Antisocial personality disorder probably predisposes both to substance misuse and psychiatric disorder. Management of DD patients should involve an integrated approach with a multidisciplinary team trained in the management of both sets of disorders, which should be treated concurrently. The use of certain PSs is socially sanctioned (e.g. opium).

As well as being obtained illicitly through drug dealers, PSs may be obtained from doctors (ostensibly therapeutically). Some may legally be bought from chemists (codeine) or shops (solvents). In the UK, some PSs (heroin, morphine, cocaine cannabis, amphetamines, barbiturates and lysergic acid diethylamide (LSD)) are controlled under the *Misuse of Drugs Act*, rendering their supply, possession, production, import or export illegal without appropriate authority/licensing. Both in the UK and USA polysubstance abuse has increased with combined use of heroin, cocaine, methadone, alcohol and tobacco.

Management involves general measures (support, rehabilitation, Drug Treatment Centres), specific antidotes (for use in overdose), medication to minimise withdrawal symptoms (e.g. benzodiazepines), and long term medication (e.g. methadone replacement for opiates or Naltrexone to neutralize opiate effects). Cognitive behavioural therapy (CBT) and related psychological approaches, such as motivational interviewing, are also used. Infection (HIV and hepatitis—especially C) is now recognized as the greatest risk associated with substance misuse; management strategies are increasingly targeted at infection risk minimization (e.g. needle exchange).

Specific substances
Opiates
Opiates include *heroin* (diamorphine; most widely used), *morphine, methadone* (Physeptone) and dextramoromide (Palfium). They may be smoked (chasing the dragon), sniffed (snorting), or taken orally, intravenously (mainlining), intramuscularly or subcutaneously (skin popping). Initially the sensation may be unpleasant (dysphoria, nausea) but this disappears with repeated usage. After an intensely pleasurable 'buzz' or 'rush', and release of histamine (itching, reddening of eyes), a sense of peace, tranquillity, detachedness occur, succeeded by CNS depression. Tolerance and withdrawal develop quickly. Ten per cent of opioid abusers become dependent but only 10% of these ever seek help for their problem; 2–3% die annually. Of the remainder 25% are abstinent at 5, and 40% at 10 years. Miosis, tremor, malaise, apathy, constipation, weakness, impotence, neglect, malnutrition and evidence of HIV and other infection are signs of chronic dependence. Early withdrawal symptoms (24–48 hours) include craving, flu-like symptoms (muscle aches, chills, rhinorrhoea, lacrimation), sweating and yawning. Mydriasis, abdominal cramps, diarrhoea, agitation, restlessness, piloerection ('gooseflesh') and tachycardia occur later (7–10 days). Symptoms may be controlled with methadone (which is less euphoriant, has a relatively long half-life and is also used for long-term maintenance), lofexidine, naltrexone or buprenorphine. Signs of overdose (often accidental) include miosis and respiratory depression and may require naloxone (opiate antagonist).

Hallucinogens
Hallucinogens include *LSD*, which produces psychological (e.g. perceptions heightened) and physiological (pupils dilated, peripheral vasoconstriction, increased temperature) effects, but not dependence. Adverse effects include 'flashbacks' (visual, occurring spontaneously for up to 1 year), schizophreniform psychoses and (in overdose) seizures. *Ecstasy* (MDMA), (a synthetic amphetamine analogue) has mixed stimulant and hallucinogenic effects and can induce hyperactivity and potentially fatal dehydration and hyperpyrexia. *Magic mushrooms* (Psylocybin) have effects similar to but less intense than LSD.

Stimulants
Amphetamines, the most commonly abused stimulants ((speed) taken orally or IV), cause euphoria, increased concentration and energy with mydriasis, tachycardia and hyperreflexia followed by depression, fatigue and headache. Chronic use may induce a schizophreniform psychosis. *Cocaine* (sympathomimetic stimulant), is sniffed (nasal ulceration), chewed or injected IV. Its effects (restlessness, increased energy, abolition of fatigue and hunger) resemble hypomania and last 20 minutes. Visual/tactile hallucinations of insects (formication), and, more rarely, paranoid psychoses occur. Post-cocaine dysphoria ('the crash') with sleeplessness and intense depression, precedes withdrawal (depression, insomnia and craving). 'Crack' (a purified and very addictive form of cocaine) is smoked. The crack 'high' is extremely short and withdrawal persecutory delusions are common.

Cannabis
The active compound of *marijuana* (pot, grass, hashish, ganja) is tetrahydrocannabinol. The effects are psychological (euphoria, relaxation, well-being, omnipotence, hallucinations) and physiological (increased appetite, lowered body temperature). No physical, but substantial psychic dependence occurs. Adverse effects include conjunctival irritation, decreased spermatogenesis, lung disease, flashbacks, transient psychoses and apathy.

Sedatives and hypnotics
Barbiturates produce relaxation and sedation, induce tolerance (NB cross tolerance with alcohol) and dependence, with withdrawal anxiety, tremor, insomnia and convulsions. Overdose may cause respiratory depression. Withdrawal is treated with BDZs or anticonvulsants. *BDZs* produce dependence, withdrawal (which may mimic the problem for which they were prescribed but may also manifest with delerium and/or seizures), and tolerance. BDZ dependence is often iatrogenic although BDZs are also common street drugs.

Others
Solvents are sniffed experimentally by groups of boys (8–19 years). Initial euphoria is followed by drowsiness. Psychological dependence is common but physical rare. Chronic abuse results in weight loss, nausea, vomiting, arrythmias, bronchospasm and cognitive impairment. Toxic effects (sometimes fatal) include hepatorenal or cerebral damage, aplastic anaemia and polyneuropathy. *Phencyclidine* (PCP, 'Angel Dust') is usually smoked. Effects include euphoria and peripheral analgesia and (in high dose) impaired consciousness or psychosis which may require antipsychotics. Withdrawal (craving, depression, retardation) may be treated with desipramine.

14 Alcohol abuse and dependence

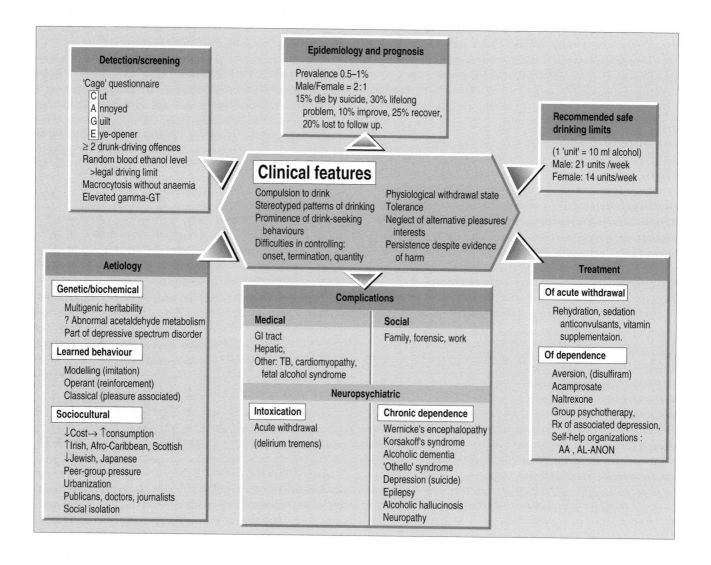

Detection/screening

'Cage' questionnaire
- **C**ut
- **A**nnoyed
- **G**uilt
- **E**ye-opener

≥ 2 drunk-driving offences
Random blood ethanol level
  >legal driving limit
Macrocytosis without anaemia
Elevated gamma-GT

Epidemiology and prognosis

Prevalence 0.5–1%
Male/Female = 2 : 1
15% die by suicide, 30% lifelong
  problem, 10% improve, 25% recover,
  20% lost to follow up.

Recommended safe drinking limits

(1 'unit' = 10 ml alcohol)
Male: 21 units /week
Female: 14 units/week

Clinical features

Compulsion to drink
Stereotyped patterns of drinking
Prominence of drink-seeking
  behaviours
Difficulties in controlling:
  onset, termination, quantity

Physiological withdrawal state
Tolerance
Neglect of alternative pleasures/
  interests
Persistence despite evidence
  of harm

Aetiology

Genetic/biochemical

Multigenic heritability
? Abnormal acetaldehyde metabolism
Part of depressive spectrum disorder

Learned behaviour

Modelling (imitation)
Operant (reinforcement)
Classical (pleasure associated)

Sociocultural

↓Cost→ ↑consumption
↑Irish, Afro-Caribbean, Scottish
↓Jewish, Japanese
Peer-group pressure
Urbanization
Publicans, doctors, journalists
Social isolation

Complications

Medical	**Social**
GI tract	Family, forensic, work
Hepatic,	
Other: TB, cardiomyopathy,	
fetal alcohol syndrome	

Neuropsychiatric

Intoxication	**Chronic dependence**
Acute withdrawal	Wernicke's encephalopathy
(delirium tremens)	Korsakoff's syndrome
	Alcoholic dementia
	'Othello' syndrome
	Depression (suicide)
	Epilepsy
	Alcoholic hallucinosis
	Neuropathy

Treatment

Of acute withdrawal

Rehydration, sedation
anticonvulsants, vitamin
supplementaion.

Of dependence

Aversion, (disulfiram)
Acamprosate
Naltrexone
Group psychotherapy,
Rx of associated depression,
Self-help organizations :
  AA , AL-ANON

Definition and clinical features

The term 'alcohol abuse' implies regular or binge consumption of alcohol sufficient to cause physical, neuropsychiatric or social damage. The conventional safe drinking limits are 21 units/week for men and 14 for women (a 'unit' of alcohol (10 ml) representing roughly a small glass of wine, a pub single of spirits or a half pint of bitter), with at least two drink-free days each week. Even much smaller amounts may be hazardous to the fetus. 'Alcohol dependence' is a syndrome with cognitive, behavioural and psychological features central to which are compulsion to drink, preoccupation with alcohol, stereotyped drinking pattern, loss of the ability to regulate drinking, altered tolerance of the intoxicant effects of alcohol (initially increased but dramatically reduced late in the disorder), withdrawal phenomena and persistence even after attempted abstinence.

Epidemiology

Prevalence rates world-wide vary widely, and are related to overall consumption levels, availability and price. The UK prevalence is ≈ 0.5–1%, with a male/female ratio of 2 : 1. Rates in women and in adolescents are increasing.

Detection and screening

Neither alcohol abuse nor dependence are always clinically obvious. Their detection is crucial not only to enable appropriate counselling and treatment and thus avoid long-term complications, but also to avoid acute withdrawal in the context of unplanned abstinence as, for example, after surgery. GPs and junior hospital staff should have a high index of suspicion in subjects with medical or psychiatric conditions associated with alcohol, and those with two or more drink/driving offences. Many cases can be identified by documenting a 'typical drinking week'. Screening questionnaires are also helpful; the simplest is the 'CAGE' (Have you felt you ought to **C**ut down your drinking? Have people **A**nnoyed you by suggesting you cut down? Have you felt **G**uilty about your drinking? Have you ever needed a drink first thing in the morning (**E**ye opener)), with one positive reply triggering further enquiry and two or more identifying problem drinking. Additional informant history can be revealing. Physical examination may reveal alcoholic stigmata, particularly signs of liver disease (spider naevi, palmar erythema, gynaecomastia) and peripheral neuropathy. Laboratory test results suggestive of problem drinking include macrocytosis without anaemia; raised gamma-GT and high blood or urine ethanol levels without obvious intoxication.

Aetiology

Aetiology is clearly multifactorial. Genetic factors have been implicated in both animal and human studies, and by the striking differences in prevalence of alcohol dependence and abuse in some racial groups (e.g. high in indigenous Americans and Australians, low in Chinese and Japanese). These may be mediated by alterations in alcohol metabolism, those at high risk producing less (hangover-causing) acetaldehyde. Heritability appears multigenic. There is often a positive family history of depression, suggesting that alcohol-related problems may form part of a genetically determined 'depressive spectrum'. Social factors include occupation (high risk in the armed forces, doctors, publicans, journalists); cultural, particularly peer-group, influences (low rates in Jews, high in Scots and Irish), and the cost of alcoholic drinks. Behavioural models stress learning by imitation (modelling), by social reinforcement (operant conditioning) and by classical conditioning (drinking to avoid withdrawal symptoms and the association between drinking and pleasure). Risk increases in the presence of chronic psychiatric or physical illness, particularly if complicated by chronic pain.

Complications

Complications include *acute intoxication*, characterized by slurred speech, impaired coordination and judgement, labile affect and, in severe cases, hypoglycaemia, stupor and coma. Differential diagnosis involves other causes of acute confusion, particularly head trauma. *Acute withdrawal* usually occurs within 1–2 days of abstinence and is characterized by malaise, nausea, autonomic hyperactivity, tremulousness, lability of mood, insomnia and transient hallucinations or illusions (usually visual). Seizures are a recognised complication. Severe withdrawal 'delirium tremens' has a mortality of up to 15%, partly as a result of other *medical complications*. These may be gastrointestinal (gastritis, peptic ulcer, pancreatitis, hepatitis, cirrhosis, oesophageal varices and/or carcinoma), haematological (anaemia, thrombocytopaenia) and cardiovascular (cardiomyopathy, hypertension). The most dramatic *neuropsychiatric complication* is Wernicke's encephalopathy (secondary to thiamine deficiency and characterized by ataxia, nystagmus, ophthalmoplegia and acute confusion), which may recover with acute administration of thiamine but develops if untreated into Korsakoff's psychosis (resolution of acute neurological signs but profound loss of short-term memory). A more generalized dementia may also occur. Other neuropsychiatric complications include peripheral neuropathy, cerebellar degeneration, alcoholic hallucinosis (usually threatening second-person voices in a clear sensorium), pathological jealousy (see pp. 78–79), symptoms of depression and/or anxiety, and erectile or ejaculatory impotence. *Social complications* include job loss, marital difficulties, criminal activity or prostitution and alcohol-related road accidents. Drinking in pregnancy may harm the fetus (*fetal alcohol syndrome*).

Management

Management of alcohol dependence needs to consider biological, psychological and social factors, and often requires a coordinated multidisciplinary and long-term approach.

The first step is to achieve abstinence and may require acute 'detoxification' which (like acute withdrawal) involves general support (adequate nutrition, reality orientation, good lighting) and measures to avoid specific complications. The latter include initially high but rapidly tailing sedation (benzodiazepines—long acting such as chlordiazepoxide or diazepam, except in liver disease) to prevent seizures and control hallucinosis (this may also require antipsychotics; haloperidol has little effect on seizure threshold); rehydration and correction of electrolyte disturbance; and B-vitamin supplementation.

Abstinence may be a more realistic long-term aim than controlled drinking. Maintenance (of abstinence or controlled drinking within safe limits) can include psychotherapy, usually in groups, aiming at sustaining motivation, learning relapse prevention strategies and developing social routines not reliant on alcohol; treatment of coexistent depression and/or anxiety; self-help groups (such as Alcoholics Anonymous); and disulfiram which blocks alcohol metabolism, inducing acetaldehyde accumulation if alcohol is ingested with resultant flushing, headache, anxiety and nausea. Acamprosate reduces craving and has recently been licenced for the maintenance of abstinence in the detoxified patient; naltrexone may have a similar effect.

Prevention involves reducing overall alcohol consumption; measures can include health education, increasing taxation on alcohol and restricting its advertising and/or sale.

Prognosis

Alcohol dependence is characterized by periods of remission and relapse; 15% of subjects die by suicide and a further 30% have lifelong alcohol-related problems. Alcohol is also often implicated in domestic violence, accidental deaths and homicides. Abuse of other drugs (particularly cross-tolerance with other sedatives such as benzodiazepines) is common. About one-third have a favourable outcome; good prognosis is more strongly associated with favourable factors in the patient (good premorbid personality, insight, motivation, family and social supports) than on any specific treatment.

15 Disorders of female reproductive life

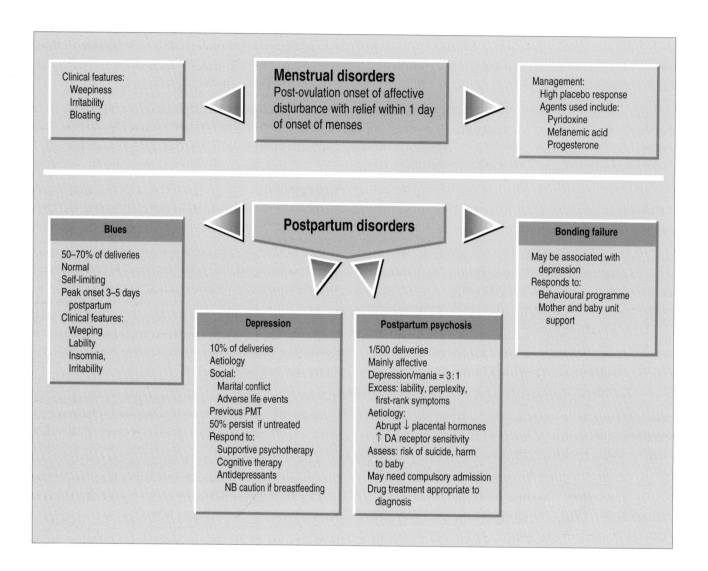

Menstrual disorders
Post-ovulation onset of affective disturbance with relief within 1 day of onset of menses

Clinical features:
Weepiness
Irritability
Bloating

Management:
High placebo response
Agents used include:
Pyridoxine
Mefanemic acid
Progesterone

Postpartum disorders

Blues
50–70% of deliveries
Normal
Self-limiting
Peak onset 3–5 days
postpartum
Clinical features:
Weeping
Lability
Insomnia,
Irritability

Bonding failure
May be associated with
depression
Responds to:
Behavioural programme
Mother and baby unit
support

Depression
10% of deliveries
Aetiology
Social:
Marital conflict
Adverse life events
Previous PMT
50% persist if untreated
Respond to:
Supportive psychotherapy
Cognitive therapy
Antidepressants
NB caution if breastfeeding

Postpartum psychosis
1/500 deliveries
Mainly affective
Depression/mania = 3 : 1
Excess: lability, perplexity,
first-rank symptoms
Aetiology:
Abrupt ↓ placental hormones
↑ DA receptor sensitivity
Assess: risk of suicide, harm
to baby
May need compulsory admission
Drug treatment appropriate to
diagnosis

The premenstrual syndrome (PMS)

PMS represents a disturbance of mood, often accompanied by other psychiatric features (insomnia, poor concentration, irritability, poor impulse control, food craving) and/or physical complaints (headache, breast tenderness and bloating). The onset is after ovulation, with rapid relief within 24 hours of the onset of menstrual flow. PMS is difficult to measure and prevalence estimates vary widely. Up to 95% of women of reproductive age have some premenstrual symptoms; up to 20% consider themselves to have PMS. Five per cent have significant psychological/physical symptoms at this time. Diagnosis is clinical by diaries of symptoms and menstruation. There is little evidence that academic performance is impaired by PMS; some studies have shown an excess of criminal activity at the end of the menstrual cycle. Possible aetiological factors include fluctuations in electrolyte and sex hormone levels, and consequent neuro-transmitter changes. Treatments include diuretics, pyridoxine, progesterone, mefanemic acid and hormonal modifications of the menstrual cycle; their evaluation is impeded by a high placebo response rate. Symptomatic treatment (including antidepressants) may also be useful.

Mental illness during pregnancy

Severe mental illness is less common in pregnancy than outside the context of childbearing; suicide in pregnancy is rare. Significant depression or anxiety occurs in about 10% of women in the first trimester; those with a past psychiatric history or with conflicting feelings about the pregnancy (such as a past or currently contemplated termination) are at particular risk. Physical treatment during pregnancy of pre-existing or emergent psychiatric conditions is problematic. Lithium and benzodiazepines are probably teratogenic; evidence regarding antidepressants and antipsychotics is equivocal. Potential benefits in individual cases must be weighed up against this risk. Caution in late pregnancy is also indicated: antipsychotics can induce an extrapyramidal syndrome in the baby and anxiolytics can cause a 'floppy baby syndrome'.

Postpartum disorders

These range from the mild, common and transient postpartum blues, through postpartum depression to the rare but florid postpartum psychoses. Risk of postpartum disorders appears similar after perinatal death (and less after abortion) to that after normal pregnancy. Adequate opportunity to grieve should be provided, however, and bereavement counselling may be required. Formal psychiatric illness following termination of pregnancy is rare, but guilt feelings are common, need ventilating and may re-emerge in subsequent pregnancies.

Postpartum blues

Postpartum blues occur after 50–70% of deliveries and should not be regarded as abnormal. The symptoms experienced are, however, sufficiently severe and out of the ordinary to warrant attention. The cardinal features are affective, with marked emotional lability, crying without external cause, irritability, sleep disturbance, and disproportionate fear of inability to cope with the baby. Onset may be at any time within the first 10 postpartum days but is typically on days 3–5. More rarely, the blues may present (usually on days 1 or 2) with elation and irritability. The aetiology remains unclear; women with a history of severe PMS (see above) are at higher risk; elevated antepartum progesterone levels and precipitate postpartum falls in oestrogen, progesterone and sodium have been implicated. No clear relationship with obstetric or social variables has been demonstrated. The blues are self-limiting, usually within a few days. No specific intervention is required (apart from reassurance), although more persistent depression must be excluded. Appropriate antenatal education, providing warning for women and their partners about the blues, is helpful.

Postpartum depression

Postpartum depression occurs in 10–15% of new mothers, with onset within the first 6 weeks after delivery. The clinical features are similar to those of depression at other times, although suicidal thoughts are less common, and preoccupation (in terms of feelings of guilt or inadequacy) with the baby is usual. Unlike the blues, postpartum depression is usually not transient; about 50% of untreated cases will still be depressed a year later. There may be persistent abnormalities of mother–child interaction. Many cases are undetected and screening for depression is an appropriate part of the 6-week postnatal check. Aetiological factors appear to be predominantly social (although a family history of depression, particularly postpartum, is common), with marital conflicts and a lack of confiding relationships particularly implicated. Management involves full social assessment (including possible risk to the baby), and treatment may include marital therapy, individual (supportive or cognitive) psychotherapy and/or antidepressants. Most antidepressants are excreted in breast milk in concentrations approximating those in maternal plasma. Fluoxetine is excreted in lower concentrations than paroxetine or tricyclics. Risks to breast-fed babies are slight but must be considered when initiating antidepressants in women keen to continue breastfeeding.

Postpartum psychoses

Postpartum psychoses occur after about one birth in 500, and usually has an abrupt onset, within 2–4 weeks after delivery. The excess is more than can be explained as a 'postponement' of such disorders from pregnancy. The clinical presentation is usually affective, the majority depressive but up to one-third with mania. Postpartum onset of schizophrenia is relatively rare, but postpartum affective psychoses are often associated with one or more Schneiderian first-rank symptoms (see Chapter 3), and are likely to show emotional lability and to be subjectively confused. The excess positive family history of affective disorder is similar to that found in bipolar patients. Risk of postpartum recurrence is at least 1/5 after one postpartum (or non-postpartum) episode, and up to 1/2 after multiple postpartum episodes. Risk appears highest in primiparae, and after instrumental delivery. Dopamine-receptor supersensitivity has been reported in high-risk subjects who subsequently develop postpartum psychoses. Management must include assessment of suicide risk and of risk to the baby, who may suffer from neglect and/or (where the mother is deluded) inappropriate care, deliberate harm or even infanticide. Treatment usually requires hospitalization, sometimes compulsorily, and where possible, with the baby to a specialist mother-and-baby unit. Drug treatment is as appropriate to the clinical presentation, although antidepressants and neuroleptics must be used with caution (and lithium is contraindicated) in breastfeeding mothers. ECT has been reported to be particularly effective, irrespective of diagnostic group. Short-term prognosis is excellent, although risk of recurrence is similar to that for non-postpartum affective disorder.

Bonding failure

Bonding failure represents the failure to develop of the normally intense emotional mother–baby bond, and may be accompanied by hostility towards the baby. It usually occurs in the context of ambivalence about the pregnancy, adverse life events and/or postpartum depression. Management, which should take place in a mother-and-baby unit, involves treatment of underlying conflicts and a combination of supportive and behavioural (modelling) psychotherapy.

Menopausal disorders

There is little evidence for specific psychiatric disorders associated with the menopause (although physical symptoms such as flushing and sweating are common) and the concept of 'involutional melancholia' has been largely discredited.

16 Functional disorders in old age

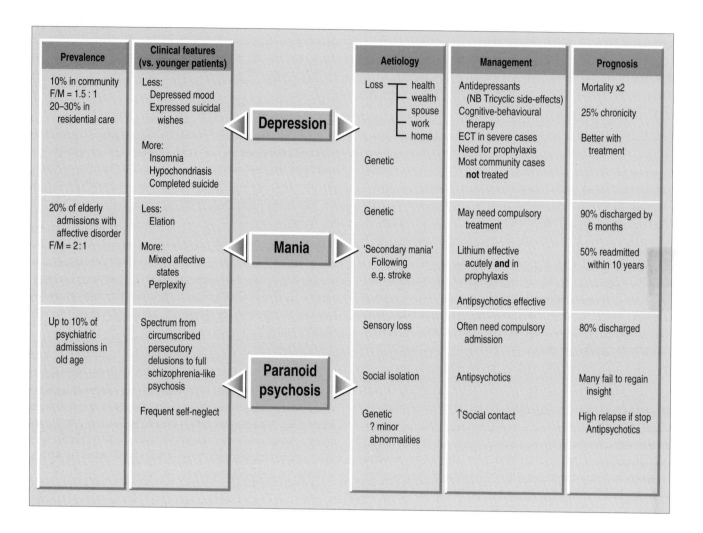

Prevalence	Clinical features (vs. younger patients)		Aetiology	Management	Prognosis
10% in community F/M = 1.5 : 1 20–30% in residential care	Less: Depressed mood Expressed suicidal wishes More: Insomnia Hypochondriasis Completed suicide	**Depression**	Loss ┬ health ├ wealth ├ spouse ├ work └ home Genetic	Antidepressants (NB Tricyclic side-effects) Cognitive-behavioural therapy ECT in severe cases Need for prophylaxis Most community cases **not** treated	Mortality x2 25% chronicity Better with treatment
20% of elderly admissions with affective disorder F/M = 2:1	Less: Elation More: Mixed affective states Perplexity	**Mania**	Genetic 'Secondary mania' Following e.g. stroke	May need compulsory treatment Lithium effective acutely **and** in prophylaxis Antipsychotics effective	90% discharged by 6 months 50% readmitted within 10 years
Up to 10% of psychiatric admissions in old age	Spectrum from circumscribed persecutory delusions to full schizophrenia-like psychosis Frequent self-neglect	**Paranoid psychosis**	Sensory loss Social isolation Genetic ? minor abnormalities	Often need compulsory admission Antipsychotics ↑Social contact	80% discharged Many fail to regain insight High relapse if stop Antipsychotics

Older people suffer from a range of functional psychiatric disorders which may present particular problems in both detection and treatment. The most important of these (depression, mania and the schizophrenia-like disorders of late life, or late paraphrenias) are discussed in turn below. Older people are also liable to experience adjustment reactions (particularly bereavement), although the presentation and management of these are essentially the same as earlier in life. In addition, they may develop anxiety disorders (both generalized and phobic). General anxiety is often either relatively mild or coexistent with (and responsive to the same treatment approaches as) depression. New phobic disorders, particularly agoraphobia, are often precipitated by traumatic events and frequently persist. Finally, older people may continue to manifest disorders of personality, although the degree of distress and disability they cause usually decreases with increasing age.

Depression in old age
Epidemiology and clinical features
Depression is about as common in late as in middle life. There is good consensus from epidemiological studies that its prevalence in late life is around 10–15%. Most studies find an overrepresentation of women (by a factor of about 1.5) and little relationship within the elderly with increasing age. The diagnosis is, however, often 'missed' in older subjects despite the fact that they frequently consult their doctor; most subjects detected in community surveys are found to be untreated. This is partly because of the unjustified idea that depression is an inevitable consequence of ageing but also because of important differences in clinical presentation. Depressed mood is less often overt in older depressed subjects, who are also less likely to express suicidal ideation despite being at substantially higher risk of completed suicide. Older depressed subjects are,

however, more likely to complain of disturbed sleep, which must be distinguished from the more insidious loss of sleep duration commonly found in normal ageing; to complain of multiple physical problems for which no cause can be found; and to exhibit motor disturbance (retardation and/or agitation). These differences in symptom pattern render conventional diagnostic criteria for depression misleading in old age, since the majority of subjects fulfil criteria for only 'minor' depression despite similar severity of illness to those with major depression and, paradoxically, a greater proportion with an 'endogenous' pattern of symptoms.

Aetiology

Genetic factors are significant, although the family history is less often positive than in younger depressed patients. In particular, subjects becoming depressed for the first time in late life often have a low genetic loading, but are more likely to have brain imaging abnormalities, cognitive impairment and poor treatment response. This suggests that late first-onset depression may, in some cases, reflect neurodegenerative change. Social isolation, particularly the lack of confiding relationships, render older people vulnerable to depression which is often triggered by the experience of loss(es) such as bereavement, deteriorating physical health or financial insecurity. Institutionalization doubles the risk of depression in old age.

Management

Both physical and psychological treatments are effective but underused in older subjects. Reducing social isolation may also be important. Cognitive and behavioural approaches may need to be modified to the needs of an older group but are effective in group as well as individual settings. Tricyclic antidepressants are as effective as in younger subjects, but their utility in practice is diminished by a higher risk of clinically important side-effects, particularly postural hypotension and resultant falls (dangerous, particularly in the presence of age-related osteoporosis which is commoner in women). Newer antidepressants such as the SSRIs may be of particular value in the elderly because of their relative lack of contraindications, safety and favourable side-effect profile. Compliance with antidepressants may be difficult to achieve in older subjects, particularly since they may take longer (up to 8 weeks) to take effect. ECT is very effective in the more severe depressions of late life, particularly in retarded and/or deluded patients and those refusing food and/or fluid in whom the risk of irreversible physical deterioration is high. MAOIs and lithium augmentation are effective in some older patients with refractory depression.

Prognosis

Depression in late life carries a mortality twice that in matched control subjects. Some of the excess is related to suicide, the risk of which is particularly high in older depressed men. There is also a high risk of chronicity (about 50% if untreated) and of relapse. The prognosis is considerably improved by early detection with appropriate acute treatment and subsequent prophylaxis; both antidepressants and lithium are effective in preventing depressive relapse.

Mania in old age

Mania in old age was thought rare but in fact accounts for about 20% of all psychiatric admissions for affective disorders in older subjects. Most subjects have a past history of depression; in about 20% the mania is precipitated by acute physical illness such as stroke. Overt elation is less often present than in mania in earlier life, although the patient generally has grandiose ideation, and the clinical picture is more usually of irritability, lability of mood and perplexity—much like that of acute confusional states which are thus the most important differential diagnoses. Antipsychotics are effective in acute treatment, although their prolonged use is to be avoided if possible because of the age-related increase in risk of tardive dyskinesia. Lithium may be used both acutely and in prophylaxis, although as many as 25% of older subjects (particularly those with Parkinson's disease or dementia) develop neurotoxicity. Both therapeutic and toxic effects of lithium may occur at lower blood levels in old age; close monitoring is therefore necessary. The prognosis with treatment is good, although recurrence occurs in up to 50% by 10 years.

Paranoid psychosis

Paranoid psychosis accounts for 10% of all psychiatric admissions in old age and represents a spectrum of presentations ranging from highly circumscribed persecutory delusions, through the presence of both delusions and hallucinations to a full-blown schizophrenia-like picture with thought disorder, passivity experiences and/or disorders of possession of thought. The debate as to whether these conditions are distinct from schizophrenia is unresolved. Acute confusional states, delusional depression and early dementia must all be considered in the differential diagnosis. Aetiological factors include a genetic component (with excess family history of psychiatric illness as a whole and particularly schizophrenia), sensory deprivation (particularly deafness) and longstanding social isolation. Brain imaging abnormalities have been reported. Treatment is often difficult because of lack of insight, but response to antipsychotics, combined if possible with social reintegration, is usually good. As older people are at particular risk of tardive dyskinesia, the use of newer, more selective dopamine blockers like Sulpiride should be first line treatment. A substantial minority never regain insight despite good functional recovery. Relapse is frequent if antipsychotics are withdrawn; this must be weighed up against the risk of tardive dyskinesia with their continued use.

17 Acute confusional states (delirium)

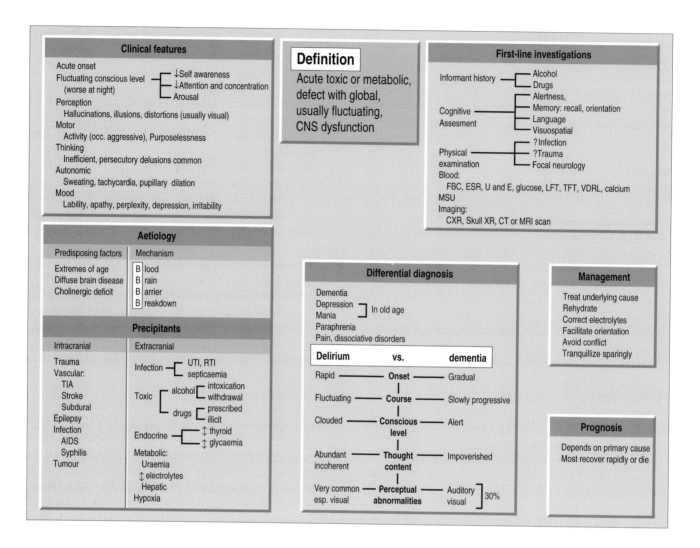

Clinical features

Acute onset
Fluctuating conscious level — ↓Self awareness
(worse at night) — ↓Attention and concentration
— Arousal
Perception
Hallucinations, illusions, distortions (usually visual)
Motor
Activity (occ. aggressive), Purposelessness
Thinking
Inefficient, persecutory delusions common
Autonomic
Sweating, tachycardia, pupillary dilation
Mood
Lability, apathy, perplexity, depression, irritability

Definition

Acute toxic or metabolic, defect with global, usually fluctuating, CNS dysfunction

First-line investigations

Informant history — Alcohol
— Drugs
Cognitive — Alertness,
Assesment — Memory: recall, orientation
— Language
— Visuospatial
Physical — ? Infection
examination — ?Trauma
— Focal neurology
Blood:
FBC, ESR, U and E, glucose, LFT, TFT, VDRL, calcium
MSU
Imaging:
CXR, Skull XR, CT or MRI scan

Aetiology

Predisposing factors	Mechanism
Extremes of age	B lood
Diffuse brain disease	B rain
Cholinergic deficit	B arrier
	B reakdown

Precipitants

Intracranial	Extracranial
Trauma	Infection — UTI, RTI
Vascular:	— septicaemia
TIA	Toxic — alcohol — intoxication
Stroke	— withdrawal
Subdural	drugs — prescribed
Epilepsy	— illicit
Infection	Endocrine — ↕ thyroid
AIDS	— ↕ glycaemia
Syphilis	Metabolic:
Tumour	Uraemia
	↕ electrolytes
	Hepatic
	Hypoxia

Differential diagnosis

Dementia
Depression ⎤ In old age
Mania ⎦
Paraphrenia
Pain, dissociative disorders

Delirium	vs.	dementia
Rapid	Onset	Gradual
Fluctuating	Course	Slowly progressive
Clouded	Conscious level	Alert
Abundant incoherent	Thought content	Impoverished
Very common esp. visual	Perceptual abnormalities	Auditory visual ⎤ 30%

Management

Treat underlying cause
Rehydrate
Correct electrolytes
Facilitate orientation
Avoid conflict
Tranquillize sparingly

Prognosis

Depends on primary cause
Most recover rapidly or die

The acute confusional state (also known as delirium) is characterized by the rapid onset of a global but fluctuating dysfunction of the CNS, with an underlying toxic, vascular, ictal or metabolic defect. It represents one of the most important problems encountered in general hospital psychiatry and is seen by a wide range of specialities including general and emergency medicine, general and orthopaedic surgery and medicine for the elderly. It may occur in as many as one-third of older patients admitted to hospital either at initial presentation or during hospitalization.

Clinical features

The most characteristic (although not inevitable) features are an acute onset of *disorientation* and *fluctuating level of consciousness* often worse at night (sundowning). The latter may involve loss of self-awareness, attention and concentration; level of arousal may be heightened or decreased. *Motor activity*

may be increased but is usually purposeless; aggressive behaviour occurs in about 10% of cases. *Mood* and affect may fluctuate rapidly (lability) and be accompanied by irritability and/or subjective perplexity; more persistent apathy or depression is also found. *Perceptual disturbances* are common. Illusions (incorrectly interpreted perceptions) are very common and often frightening; true hallucinations are also common, most frequently visual and usually simple (e.g. geometric patterns or ill-defined shapes). Real objects may appear distorted with size apparently increased or decreased (macro-/micropsia). *Thinking* is inefficient; patients complain of being slow and muddled; speech is sometimes incoherent. Poorly systematized, transient delusions are common; these may be secondary to abnormal perceptions and are often persecutory with associated ideas of reference. Sweating, tachycardia and dilated pupils reflect underlying autonomic overactivity.

Aetiology

Predisposing factors

Delirium is commonest in the very young and the very old. Those with diffuse brain disease (such as dementia or Parkinson's disease) are particularly vulnerable, as are those with deficits in cholinergic neurotransmission or taking drugs with anticholinergic properties (e.g. tricyclic antidepressants, procyclidine). Breakdown of the blood–brain barrier is thought to be fundamental. *Precipitants* may be classified as *intracranial* and *extracranial*. Among the former are trauma (e.g. boxing injury) and vascular insults including stroke and haemorrhage (particularly in the subdural space where the presentation may be subacute, and extradurally where sudden collapse may occur after a 'lucid interval'). Epilepsy and intracranial tumour may also present with acute confusion, as may intracranial infection (meningitis, encephalitis or abscess). The great cerebral masqueraders (TB, neurosyphilis, AIDS) must always be considered. A wide range of extracranial pathology can result in delirium. Infective causes include urinary tract infection (UTI), pneumonia (which may be 'silent' in old age) and septicaemia. Toxic reactions to drugs frequently cause confusion. Prescribed drugs (including antidepressants, tranquillizers and diuretics) may accumulate in the elderly. Alcohol may confuse both through intoxication (tolerance often decreasing with age) and, most importantly, through withdrawal (delirium tremens (the DTs)). Delirium tremens may occur following abrupt alcohol withdrawal in the context of elective or emergency hospitalization, emphasizing the importance of an accurate alcohol history. Endocrine and metabolic causes of delirium include thyroid hyper- and hypofunction, hyper- and hypoglycaemia (the latter usually more dramatic in onset) and failure of major body systems (heart, lungs, liver, kidneys). Hypoxia is a frequent final common pathway. Nutritional causes (B_1, B_{12} or folate deficiency) are uncommon, except when secondary to alcohol abuse. In this context, acute B_1 deficiency (Wernicke's encephalopathy, characterized by ataxia, ophthalmoplegia, nystagmus and confusion) represents a medical emergency since, if untreated, irreversible brain damage (Korsakoff's psychosis characterized by short-term memory loss and confabulation) occurs.

Differential diagnosis

Conditions resembling delirium include chronic confusional states (dementias), functional psychiatric conditions (in the elderly both mania and depression as well as paraphrenia should be considered), and responses to major stress, particularly severe pain and dissociative disorders. The diagnosis depends on the demonstration of the cardinal features of delirium (particularly fluctuation in both conscious level and cognitive impairment), the presence of a specific underlying cause and the lack of *consistent* features of affective or psychotic disorders. The differentiation between delirium and dementia may be difficult, since people with established dementia are particularly vulnerable to delirium. Delirium should be considered where deterioration has been rapid, the course is fluctuating (rather than slowly progressive), consciousness is clouded rather than alert, and thought content (which in dementia is usually impoverished) is vivid, complex and muddled. Hallucinations occur both in delirium and dementia. In delirium they are very common and predominantly visual; in dementia, on the other hand, they are as frequently auditory and are only found in about one-third of cases.

Investigations

It is imperative to obtain an informant history, focusing particularly on premorbid level of functioning, onset and course of the confusion and use/abuse of drugs or alcohol. In the mental state assessment, particular attention should be paid to cognitive function (alertness, memory, language, visuospatial ability) and to fluctuation in behaviour. Physical examination is crucial in identifying focal neurological signs and/or evidence of infection or trauma. Essential blood tests include FBC (to exclude anaemia, macrocytosis, leucocytosis), erythrocyte sedimentation rate (ESR) (infection), U and E (dehydration, electrolyte imbalance), glucose, thyroid and liver function tests, calcium and VDRL. MSU is mandatory and chest and skull X-rays may be informative. Structural brain imaging (CT or MRI) and EEG, where available, can identify many intracranial causes.

Management

Specific management should be targeted at detection of the confusional state itself, and at identification and subsequent treatment of underlying pathology. General management includes facilitation of orientation. Patients should be nursed in a quiet well-lit room, avoiding frequent changes in staff. Patients may be very anxious and require consistent explanation and reassurance. Dehydration and electrolyte imbalance are common irrespective of underlying cause and must be corrected. Aggressive outbursts may be minimized by reassurance and the anticipation and avoidance of potential conflict. Where undesirable behaviour must be controlled, antipsychotics are preferable to physical restraint but should be used sparingly; hypotensive and anticholinergic side-effects may precipitate falls or exacerbate the confusion. Haloperidol is the drug of choice, except when the patient is withdrawing from alcohol or drug abuse, where diazepam is more suitable.

Prognosis

Mortality is high, although dependent on the underlying cause and reduced by rapid diagnosis, identification of any underlying pathology and appropriate general and specific treatment. Where recovery occurs it is usually rapid, with return to premorbid functional level.

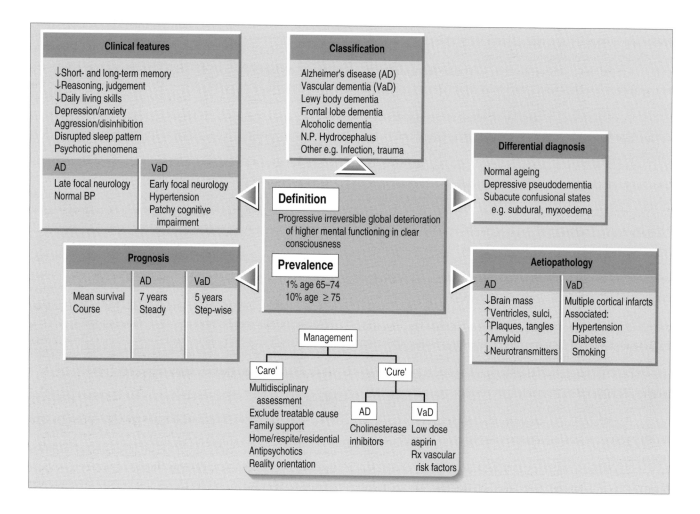

Definition and clinical presentation

Dementia is a syndrome rather than a diagnosis. The term refers to a global deterioration of higher mental functioning in clear consciousness that is progressive and (usually) irreversible. The most obvious manifestations are disruption of memory (long as well as short term), of language (nominal aphasia being particularly common) and of 'intelligence' in terms of reasoning, judgement and performance in IQ tests. Other features include changes in personality and in behaviour, as reflected both in loss of daily living skills (such as washing and dressing or handling money) and in abnormal behaviours, including aggression, wandering and sexual disinhibition. Apathy, depression and anxiety are frequent and there may be disturbances of sleep, including daytime drowsiness, confusion between day and night and nocturnal restlessness. Psychotic phenomena, particularly persecutory delusions (aggravated by forgetfulness) and auditory or visual hallucinations occur in about one-third of subjects. Dementia interferes with the sufferer's family, work and social functioning. Presentation seldom occurs until the dementia has

been present for at least 1 year and is often at the instigation of a worried family member. The clinical presentation may differ between types of dementia (see Classification below).

Epidemiology

Dementia becomes commoner with increasing age. Onset before the age of 65 is very rare but 1% of the population aged 65–74 are affected as are 10% of those aged 75+ and 25% of those aged 85+. As the 'very old' population in the developed world increases, the absolute number of those with dementia will rise much more steeply as will the family, social and financial burdens of providing adequate dementia care.

Classification

The major dementias are degenerative. These include Alzheimer's disease (AD, about 50% of cases) and the vascular dementias (such as vascular dementia, VaD—20–30% of cases, including those with a 'mixed' AD/VaD picture). VaD is associated with more patchy cognitive impairment than AD, focal neurological symptoms or signs and a 'stepwise' rather than continuous deterioration. A recently described dementia, Dementia with Lewy bodies (DLB), characterized by fluctuating cognitive functioning, visual hallucinations, sensitivity to neuroleptic side-effects and Parkinsonian features may account for as many as 20% of people with dementia. Dementia in the context of chronic alcohol abuse accounts for up to 10% of cases. More rarely, dementia may be associated with repeated head trauma (as in boxers) or infection (HIV, syphilis, prion). Normal pressure hydrocephalus (NPH) may be idiopathic or due to subarachnoid haemorrhage, head injury or meningitis. NPH produces a 'patchy' dementia with marked mental slowness, apathy and early onset of gait abnormalities and loss of control of micturition. Ventriculo-atrial shunting may benefit up to 50% of cases.

Aetiopathology

1 Alzheimer's Disease. At macroscopic level (and on CT or MRI scan), the brain in AD is shrunken, with increased sulcal widening and enlarged ventricles. Microscopically, the key changes are neuronal loss, and the presence (particularly in cortex and hippocampus) of 'amyloid plaques' (containing a core of amyloid protein) and neurofibrillary tangles. Neurochemically, there are deficits in several neurotransmitters including acetylcholine, noradrenaline, serotonin and somatostatin, with corresponding loss of the cell bodies of neurons secreting these transmitters. A number of specific abnormalities have recently been found in genes coding for the protein precursor of amyloid; most relate to rare familial forms of AD, however, one genetic polymorphism, in the Apolipoprotein E gene, may be a clinically useful market of risk in subjects with late onset, non-familial AD. Three common alleles (E2, E3, E4) exist; the E4 allele (particularly if homozygous) appears to indicate increased risk and risk of relatively early onset. Other aetiological factors include poor education and damage by free radicals. Hormone replacement therapy may protect against AD in women. The next few years are likely to see further progress in elucidating the multifactorial 'cascade' leading from the formation of abnormal amyloid precursor protein to AD.

2 Vascular or multi-infarct dementia (VaD) is associated with multiple areas of cortical infarction, with volume of infarction more crucial than infarct location in determining progression to dementia. Damage to deep white matter vasculature may also cause a dementia. In both cases, the primary pathology usually involves vascular factors such as stroke, hypertension, heart disease, diabetes and smoking.

3 Dementia with Lewy bodies (DLB) is associated with the presence in cerebral cortex of Lewy bodies identical to those found in the basal ganglia in Parkinson's disease. Pathological changes characteristic of AD are also often found.

4 Frontal lobe dementias including Pick's disease are characterized by early personality changes and relative intellectual sparing.

Differential diagnosis

Many normal elderly people develop mild, circumscribed deterioration in memory or 'age-associated memory impairment'; they may need reassurance that they do not have a dementia. Severe depression in old age may present with a 'pseudodementia' with prominent forgetfulness and poor self-care. Such patients, unlike those with a true dementia, usually have a short history and are often aware of, and distressed by, their poor function. Acute confusional states, particularly where only slowly progressive (e.g. subdural haematoma, myxoedema and vitamin deficiencies) may present with a dementia-like picture.

Management

There is currently no 'cure' for AD, VaD or DLB, although there may be some functional improvement in patients with VaD in whom vascular risk factors for stroke are controlled; low-dose aspirin also reduces risk of further stroke-related deterioration. Cholinesterase inhibitors (donepezil, rivastigmine) may improve both cognition and behaviour in mild to moderate AD. Patients should have a full multidisciplinary assessment to exclude treatable causes and identify specific problems. The possibility of superadded and treatable acute confusional states (commonly iatrogenic or secondary to infection) should always be considered if a patient deteriorates. Depression often complicates established dementia and may respond to antidepressants.

The focus of management of dementia must be on care delivery, assessing and responding to the changing needs of affected patients and their family carers, and maintaining dignity and individuality. Support may include home-care input as well as day and intermittent respite in social service or hospital settings. Patients with severe dementia may require residential, nursing home or (where behavioural problems are prominent) hospital care. Behavioural problems may respond to low-dose antipsychotics. Psychological techniques such as reality orientation may also improve cognition and behaviour. There is likely to be considerable progress in the next 10–20 years in developing disease modification strategies: in AD these may include neuro protective agents such as antioxidants, drugs to prevent amyloid formation and gene therapies.

Prognosis

Patients with AD usually deteriorate inexorably to an endstage needing full nursing care; death is often from bronchopneumonia (although very elderly patients frequently die of other causes before the dementia becomes severe). Mean life expectancy is 7 years from diagnosis. VaD has a slightly worse prognosis; progression is less consistent with vulnerability to sudden stroke-related death. Skilled nursing care may substantially increase life expectancy in very severe dementia.

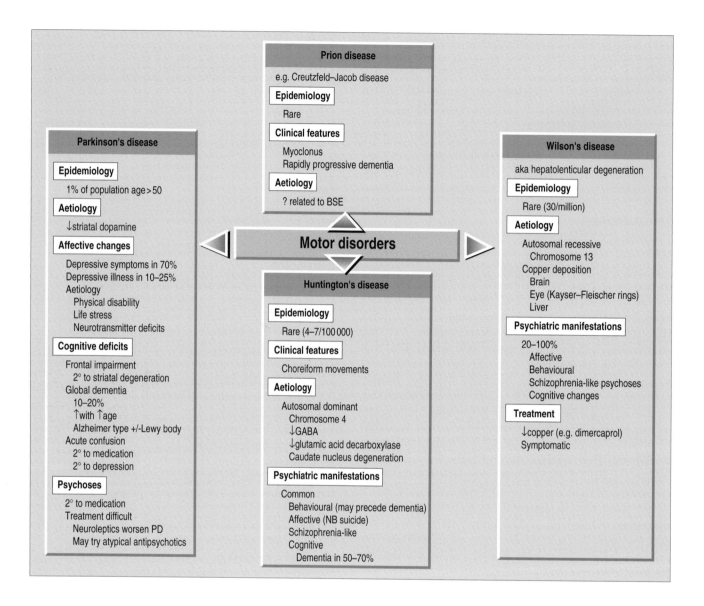

Neuropsychiatry is primarily concerned with those conditions in which mental disorder results from demonstrable structural or neurophysiological disturbance of the brain. There are several ways of classifying these disorders, including focal and diffuse, specific and global and according to aetiology. Cerebral causes include degenerative (dementias, Parkinson's disease, Huntington's disease), infections (syphilis, AIDS), epilepsy and miscellaneous (multiple sclerosis, Wilson's disease). Systemic causes include metabolic disturbances (e.g. porphyria), endocrinopathies and vitamin deficiencies.

In general, the psychiatric aspects of organic disorders may be divided into personality and behavioural changes, cognitive difficulties, affective disturbances, psychoses and drug-induced problems, e.g. confusional states. The psychiatric picture seldom bears a specific relationship to the type of underlying pathology, being more influenced by the site of brain involvement and the time course of the illness. The presentation is also coloured by the patient's premorbid personality, predisposition to psychiatric disorder and social circumstances. An organic disorder can mimic functional disorders, but points in favour of organic problems include cognitive disorder preceding mood or other disorder, specific cognitive deficits, neurological signs, fluctuating symptomatology, visual hallucinations, vague or transient paranoid delusions, and symptoms not typical of a functional disorder. In order to make the diagnosis, a full psychiatric history and mental state examination (see Chapter 1), and full physical and neurological examinations must be undertaken. Special investigations should include a general screen (see Chapter 17). Where a specific diagnosis is suspected, more specific investigations (as detailed under individual conditions below) may help in its confirmation. Lumbar puncture should be undertaken with caution if raised intracranial pressure is suspected in view of the risk of precipitating brainstem coning.

Dementias are sometimes classified as cortical or subcortical, although neither type exclusively affects only cortical or subcortical tissue. Subcortical dementias include Parkinson's Disease, Huntingdon's Disease and Progressive Supra–Nuclear palsy. Symptoms include psychomotor slowing and executive dysfunction associated with disruption to frontal pathways, in addition to disease–specific symptoms. Subcortical dementias are rarely associated with focal cognitive symptoms such as aphasia or agnosia.

Parkinson's disease

Parkinson's disease (PD), affecting over 1% of the population above 50 years of age, results from deficient striatal dopaminergic activity. Psychiatric disturbances are common and include intellectual impairment, affective changes and psychoses. Global dementia occurs in 10–20% of PD patients over 65 years (AD and DLB), with increasing age being an important contributory factor. Frontal lobe cognitive deficits are seen early in PD and relate to striatal dysfunction. Isolated focal abnormalities (e.g. immediate recall of verbal material, working memory), drug-induced confusional states (especially with antimuscarinic compounds and selegiline) and depression-related cognitive difficulties are also common. Affective disturbances (depressive symptoms (70%), depressive illness (10–25%)) may be confounded by physical symptoms of PD and are complex in aetiology, with both neurotransmitter systems (dopaminergic, serotonergic, cholinergic) and social problems (low self-esteem, physical disability, poorly targeted coping strategies, dissatisfaction with support, social stress, sexual problems) being invoked. The degree of motor disability does not correlate strongly with abnormalities of mood, although depression may be encountered more often in patients with prominent gait and postural changes. Treatment of depression and psychoses should, where possible, be with drugs less liable to induce neurological side-effects to which such patients are particularly vulnerable. Atypical antipsychotics may be useful as they are associated with a low incidence of extrapyramidal side-effects.

Huntington's disease

Huntington's disease (HD), characterized by choreiform involuntary movements and 'fidgetiness', is inherited as an autosomal dominant gene (100% penetrance) on the short arm of chromosome 4. Rare individuals have a negative family history which may be due to a new spontaneous mutation or illegitimacy. HD manifests at 25–50 years of age, affects males and females equally and prevalence is 4–7/100 000. There is cerebral atrophy, reduced gamma-aminobutyric acid (GABA) and GAD, resulting in dopamine hypersensitivity (especially caudate and putamen). Psychiatric disturbances, common in both individuals at risk and in patients with HD, include changes in behaviour/personality (apathy, irritability), affective disorders (depression = 40%; mania = 10%), and schizophreniform psychoses as well as cognitive impairment or frank dementia (50–70% of patients with chorea). The dementia is subcortical, characterized by poor cognitive function, mental slowing and a decline in memory, but no dysfunction of language and no focal deficits of perception. Many patients with HD have insight into their intellectual impairment (which may precede other symptoms). Depression can also precede other symptoms and occurs in a subset of families. Suicide occurs both in patients with HD and in those at risk, and must be borne in mind when planning genetic counselling and predictive testing. Treatment for HD is symptomatic, and depression and psychoses should be treated with standard medications. Death occurs about 15 years after diagnosis.

Hepatolenticular degeneration

Hepatolenticular degeneration also known as Wilson's disease (WD) is an uncommon inborn error of metabolism (estimated at 30/million) transmitted by an autosomal recessive gene (mapped to chromosome 13) and characterized by an accumulation of copper in liver, brain, kidney, cornea (Kayser–Fleischer rings) and bone. WD is characterized by abnormal movements (e.g. generalized tremor, dystonia), muscular rigidity, dysarthria, dysphagia and cirrhosis of the liver. Psychiatric manifestations occur in 20–100% and may be the presenting feature. The most common psychiatric symptom clusters are affective (e.g. emotional lability, irritability, incongruity, anxiety, depression, mania) and behavioural changes (e.g. aggressive, antisocial). Schizophrenia-like psychoses are uncommon. Cognitive changes are well recognized (deficits in memory, visuospatial and learning skills, learning disability, dementia) and occur in those with neurological rather than hepatic impairment and with abnormalities of the basal ganglia on CT scan. Treatment is with 'anticopper drugs' (e.g. dimercaprol, penicillamine, trientine); psychiatric disturbances are treated with antidepressants or antipsychotics.

Human forms of *spongiform encephalopathy* (prion disorders e.g. Creutzfeld–Jacob disease (CJD)), are characterized by accumulation of an abnormal form of a normal host protease-resistant protein (PrP) in the brain. They present with a rapidly fatal dementia associated with myoclonic jerks. CJD is familial (15%; sometimes autosomal dominant) and the incidence is 1/million per year. These disorders also occur in animals, e.g. bovine spongiform encephalopathy (BSE—'mad cow disease') and scrapie. A link has been established between BSE and 'new form', early onset, human CJD.

20 Neuropsychiatry II

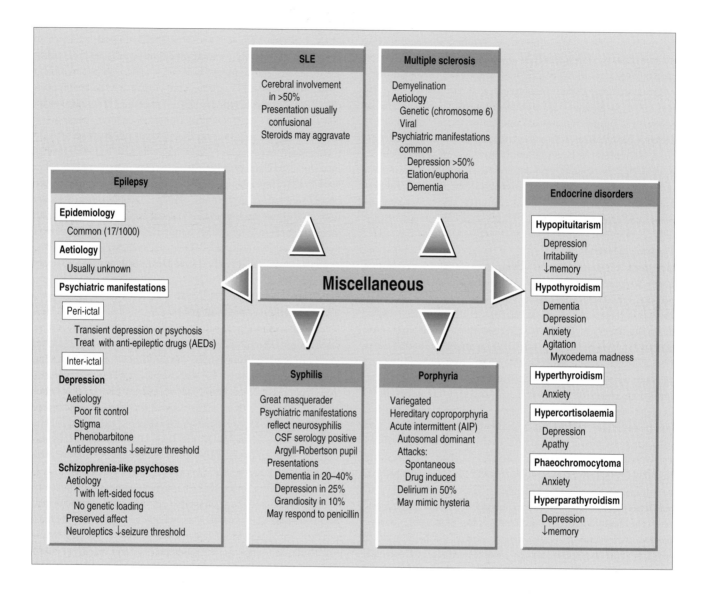

Epilepsy

Epilepsy is common (lifetime prevalence = 17/1000; prevalence of active epilepsy = 5/1000), affecting males more. Age at onset is usually before 30 years (75%), the commonest seizure type being complex partial (60%), 90% arising in temporal lobes. Aetiology is unknown in the majority of cases (75%). Psychiatric aspects of epilepsy may be divided into peri-ictal (relating to the ictus or seizures) and interictal (disturbances are chronic and not related to the ictal electric discharge). Depression is common in people with epilepsy (PWE), the commonest and clinically relevant entity being interictal depression. Mania and elation are rare. Depression, which may be severe and rapid in onset, is more likely to occur in patients with temporal lobe epilepsy (TLE)/complex partial seizures (CPS), of whom

20% become depressed. There may be a decrease in seizure frequency prior to the depression and a predominance of left-sided lesions. Other neuroepilepsy variables (e.g. age of onset of epilepsy, presence of an intracranial lesion) do not seem related to depression. Aetiological factors include antiepileptic drugs (AEDs), (e.g. phenobarbitone (PB) and vigabatrin), genetic predisposition, gender (possibly males more) and psychosocial factors (adverse life events, poor adjustment to seizures, social stigmatization, financial stress, unemployment). Suicide is increased in PWE (5× general population; TLE 25×). Treatment includes AED monotherapy (e.g. carbamazepine (improves mood) if possible), careful use of antidepressants as most (except MAOIs) lower the seizure threshold (SSRIs possibly better) and ECT if necessary. There is an increased incidence of schizophrenia-like psychoses (usually paranoid) in PWE. The psychoses (which usually develop after a latent period of 10–15 years after onset of epilepsy) are associated with left TLE, neurological abnormalities, negative family history of schizophrenia and a 'warm' affect with little personality deterioration. Treatment is with antipsychotics which lower the seizure threshold less than other AEDs, e.g. haloperidol. Cognitive changes are common in PWE and may be caused by AEDs (PB, phenytoin) or persistent abnormal electrical activity in the brain between seizures. Pseudo-seizures simulate real seizures and often occur in patients who have true seizures. They are often frequent, occur when others are present, indoors or at home, have an emotional precipitant and are associated with a history of childhood sexual abuse. Characteristically, the EEG (during the attack) and the serum prolactin (after the attack) are normal. Most PWE have a normal personality and when a personality disorder does occur it is not of any particular kind. Sexual dysfunction is common in PWE (causes include the effect of AEDs, neurophysiological problems (more common in TLE) and social problems).

Multiple sclerosis

Multiple sclerosis (MS) is common and characterized by episodes of demyelination which result in CNS abnormalities disseminated in time and space. Both genetics (chromosome 6 possibly responsible) and environment (e.g. virus) are aetiologically important. Psychiatric manifestations include personality changes, elation/euphoria (often associated with cognitive impairment), depression (>50%), suicide, cognitive impairment (early on) and progressive dementia (late stages). Denial of disability is common.

Syphilis

Syphilis (treponema pallidum infection) has three stages: primary (chancre at the site of inoculation), secondary (cutaneous rashes, condylomata, mucous patches, lymphadenopathy) and tertiary (rare today but including meningovascular and parenchymatous (optic atrophy, general paralysis of the insane (GPI), tabes dorsalis) subtypes). Positive CSF serology and raised CSF protein (neurosyphilis) occurs in the tertiary stage, may be asymptomatic or can present with any type of psychiatric symptomatology. Meningovascular syphilis appears 1–5 years after the primary infection and can present with headache, malaise, lethargy, irritability, delirium or dementia. Tabes dorsalis, appearing 8–12 years after the primary infection, presents with lightning pains, ataxia, paraesthesias and Argyll-Robertson pupils (small, irregular, reactive to convergence but not to light). GPI, appearing 5–25 years after the primary infection, has an insidious onset. There may be personality (disinhibition, irritability, lability) and cognitive (poor concentration) changes, dementia (20–40%), depression (25%), grandiosity (10%) and, more rarely, mania and schizophrenia-like psychoses. Intramuscular penicillin remains the first-line treatment and may induce neuropsychiatric improvement even in advanced disease.

Porphyria

Porphyria consists of three types: acute intermittent porphyria (AIP), hereditary coproporphyria and variegate porphyria; all are rare. AIP is a metabolic error of haem breakdown which leads to porphobilinogen in urine, is transmitted by an autosomal dominant gene with variable penetrance and is slightly more common in females (F/M = 3 : 2). AIP is characterized by acute attacks which may occur spontaneously or be precipitated by drugs (barbiturates, sulphonamides, methyldopa, oral contraception, hypoglycaemics, alcohol), infections, pregnancy, metabolic and nutritional factors (e.g. low carbohydrate intake). Clinical presentation may be abdominal (colicky pain, vomiting, constipation) and neurological (peripheral neuropathy, bulbar palsies, epilepsy). Psychiatric disturbances are found more often in AIP than in any other form of porphyria and include delirium (50%), depression, emotional lability, schizophrenia-like psychoses (especially paranoid) and symptoms incorrectly diagnosed as 'hysteria'. It has been claimed that the psychiatric disorders of King George III were manifestations of porphyria.

Systemic Lupus Erythematosus

Systemic lupus erythematosus (SLE) is a connective tissue disorder which can present with skin changes, renal involvement, arthritis and cerebral SLE (>50%). Characteristically, there are transient, fluctuating psychiatric disturbances of which the acute organic reaction is commonest. Depressive psychosis may occur less frequently and schizophrenia-like psychoses are rare. Treatment with steroids may cause further psychiatric complications.

Endocrine

Endocrine causes of psychiatric symptoms include pituitary, thyroid, adrenal and parathyroid abnormalities. Hypopituitarism (Simmond's disease) is almost invariably associated with depression, irritability and/or impaired memory. Hypothyroidism may present as dementia, depression, anxiety or acute agitation (myxoedema madness—with features of predominantly agitated depression). Hyperthyroidism can be associated with anxiety or depression (which may be delusional). Hypercortisolaemia, which is most commonly iatrogenic, may induce depression or mania. Hypocortisolaemia (Addison's disease) is usually associated with depression and apathy. Phaeochromocytoma may present with episodic anxiety accompanied by labile hypertension. Hyperparathyroidism is often accompanied by depression and apathy and occasionally by memory deficits.

Vitamin B$_{12}$

Vitamin B$_{12}$ deficiency results in pernicious anaemia and may be accompanied by subacute combined degeneration of the spinal cord associated with signs of neuropathy and spinal cord involvement. Psychiatric symptoms include slowing of mental processes, confusion, memory problems, intellectual impairment (all associated with low serum B$_{12}$), depression and paranoid delusions. Treatment is with hydroxycobalamin.

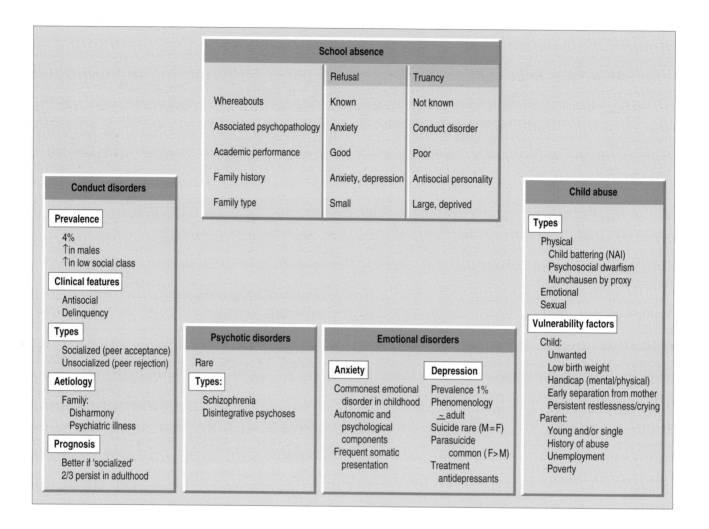

School absence

	Refusal	Truancy
Whereabouts	Known	Not known
Associated psychopathology	Anxiety	Conduct disorder
Academic performance	Good	Poor
Family history	Anxiety, depression	Antisocial personality
Family type	Small	Large, deprived

Conduct disorders

Prevalence

4%
↑in males
↑in low social class

Clinical features

Antisocial
Delinquency

Types

Socialized (peer acceptance)
Unsocialized (peer rejection)

Aetiology

Family:
 Disharmony
 Psychiatric illness

Prognosis

Better if 'socialized'
2/3 persist in adulthood

Psychotic disorders

Rare

Types:

Schizophrenia
Disintegrative psychoses

Emotional disorders

Anxiety

Commonest emotional
 disorder in childhood
Autonomic and
 psychological
 components
Frequent somatic
 presentation

Depression

Prevalence 1%
Phenomenology
 ≈ adult
Suicide rare (M=F)
Parasuicide
 common (F>M)
Treatment
 antidepressants

Child abuse

Types

Physical
 Child battering (NAI)
 Psychosocial dwarfism
 Munchausen by proxy
Emotional
Sexual

Vulnerability factors

Child:
 Unwanted
 Low birth weight
 Handicap (mental/physical)
 Early separation from mother
 Persistent restlessness/crying
Parent:
 Young and/or single
 History of abuse
 Unemployment
 Poverty

Psychiatric assessment of children

The assessment will involve interview(s) with the child and with informants (usually parents and a teacher). The informant history must cover the presenting problem (nature, precipitants, alleviators, effect on family), other current behavioural or emotional difficulties (including mood, sleep, appetite, elimination, relationships and antisocial behaviours), school behaviour and academic performance, daily routine (including hobbies), personal history (pregnancy, milestones, past illnesses/injuries/ hospitalizations, abuse, etc.) and family structure and function (parental characteristics, quality of parenting, family interactions, past or current separations). Direct assessment of the child's behaviour will focus on his/her appearance (including signs of neglect or injury), nature and level of spontaneous activity, affect, rapport with interviewer, interaction with parent(s), mannerisms and psychotic features. Physical examination, including neurological screening, is an important element of the initial assessment.

Classification

The classification of child psychiatric disorders is broadly divided into conduct disorders and emotional disorders (which may coexist), developmental disorders (pervasive or specific), disorders of elimination, hyperkinetic disorders, psychotic disorders, psychiatric aspects of child abuse and disorders of sleep.

Conduct (behavioural) disorders

These are characterized by persistent antisocial behaviours, such as disobedience, lying, truancy, aggression, stealing, promiscuity and damage to property (including firesetting). The prevalence is 4% with a male/female ratio of 3 : 1 and a marked lower social class preponderance. Low self-esteem and poor peer relationships are present in 20%; these are classified as 'mixed' conduct/emotional disorders. The term 'delinquency' refers to the subgroup who break the law. Conduct disorders may be classified into 'socialized' (where the antisocial behaviours are viewed as normal within the peer group and/or family) and 'unsocialized' where the antisocial behaviour is solitary and associated with peer and parental rejection. Aetiological factors include family disharmony, with frequent parental violence, aggression, alcoholism, antisocial personality disorder and depression. Conduct disorder is linked strongly to educational failure, especially specific reading retardation. Management usually involves a combination of family therapy, behavioural treatment of aggression and remedial teaching as well as the provision of alternative peer group activities. Antisocial behaviours persist into adult life in two-thirds; the prognosis is better in the 'socialized' group.

Emotional disorders

These are present in 2–3% of children with a female preponderance and a generally favourable prognosis. The major subtypes are described below; recent classificatory systems have proposed additional categories including social sensitivity, separation anxiety, hypochondriasis, conversion disorders, and sibling rivalry. In general, treatment involves a combination of behavioural and family therapy.

School refusal (or school phobia) accounts for 1% of school absences, with no gender or social class differences and peaks at ages 5 and 11. The presentation may be with somatic symptoms (headache, abdominal pain). Three categories are recognized: separation anxiety (younger children); fear of a specific aspect of school or travel; and low self-esteem which may in turn reflect an underlying depression. Parents (often overprotective with no excess of marital discord) are aware and often collude. Treatment is aimed at graded or abrupt resumption of school attendance. Outcome is good in 60%, although one-third have neurotic disorders in adulthood.

Generalized anxiety, the most common emotional disorder in childhood, has both physical (palpitations, dry mouth) and psychological (fear) components. Somatic symptoms, particularly abdominal pain, are also common. Predisposing factors include the child's temperament and parental overprotection.

Phobias, particularly of the dark or of strangers, are common in small children and usually are not clinically significant. When persistent and intense (often in response to parental or social reinforcement) the consequent avoidance may become pathological.

Depression is characterized, as in adults, by pervasively low mood, anhedonia, altered sleep and appetite, depressive cognitions, including reduced self-esteem, and self-destructive thoughts. It is distinguished by severity and persistence from normal sadness and it should be noted that fleeting suicidal thoughts are quite common in healthy pre-adolescents. Recent evidence (using structured clinical interviews) suggests a prevalence for depression of 1% in pre-pubertal children. Exceptionally in the context of child psychiatry, drug treatment (antidepressants) is an important component of treatment. Completed suicide is rare in children, equal in boys and girls and

there is no particular class distribution. Attempted suicide is more common, girls attempting three times more than boys, and has a higher incidence in lower socio-economic classes.

Bereavement reactions are common and characterized by prolonged sadness, irritability, guilt and crying which may last for several months with similar stages of grief to those experienced by adults. Enuresis and temper tantrums may be precipitated in younger children, while in older children sleep disturbance, poor school performance and depressive illness may ensue. The surviving parent's coping mechanisms are crucial.

Obsessive-compulsive disorder (OCD) is rare in early childhood (prevalence 0.3%), although isolated compulsions (not walking on paving stone lines) are common. OCD presents much as in adults and usually responds to a combination of behavioural methods (usually requiring family cooperation) and serotonin-focused antidepressants.

Child abuse

The concept covers neglect and emotional abuse as well as sexual and/or physical assault (including non-accidental injury). Abuse can occur in all social strata and a high index of suspicion is crucial. Vulnerability factors in the child include being unwanted, having a low birth weight, early maternal separation, mental or physical handicap and persistent restlessness or crying. Young and/or single parents with their own history of abuse, adverse socio-economic circumstances (particularly unemployment), and unrealistic styles of disciplining are particularly liable to abuse their children. Signs of abuse include injuries without convincing explanation, previous history of similar injury, and evidence in the child of withdrawal and/or fear of parents. Emotional abuse is an important cause of non-organic 'failure to thrive'. Psychiatric consequences of child abuse include increased vulnerability to subsequent emotional, conduct and developmental disorders later in childhood, as well as depression, conversion disorders (e.g. pseudo-seizures) and childrearing problems in adult life. Management involves detection, confrontation, arranging protection for the child if necessary, and individual and family therapy.

Sleep problems

These are common in normal children with restless sleep in 30%, night-time wakefulness in 20% and sleeptalking in 10%. Night terrors, in which children sit up terrified and screaming but cannot be woken sufficiently to be reassured, have a peak incidence (3%) at age 4–7 and a frequently positive family history. They arise from deep (stage 4) sleep and are accompanied by tachycardia and tachypnoea. They are aggravated by daytime stress and usually resolve spontaneously. Nightmares (peak incidence 5 to 6 years) may be equally frightening and are also often stress related; the child can, however, be easily woken and reassured.

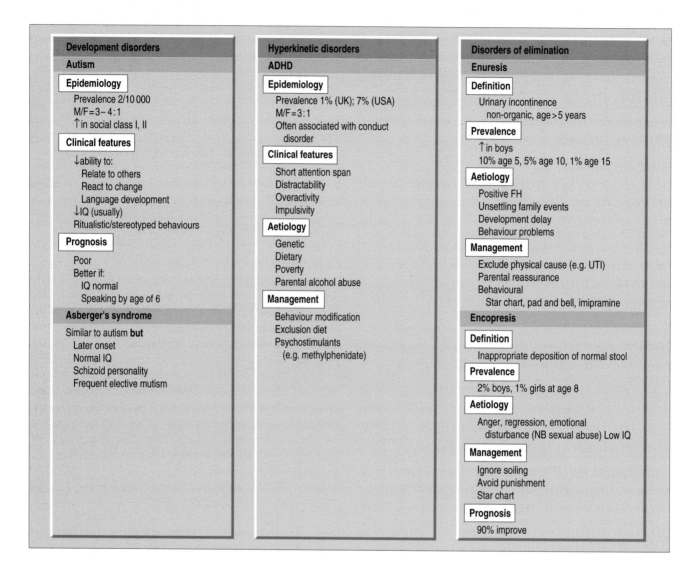

Development disorders	Hyperkinetic disorders	Disorders of elimination
Autism	**ADHD**	**Enuresis**
Epidemiology	Epidemiology	Definition
Prevalence 2/10 000 M/F = 3 – 4 : 1 ↑in social class I, II	Prevalence 1% (UK); 7% (USA) M/F = 3 : 1 Often associated with conduct disorder	Urinary incontinence non-organic, age > 5 years
Clinical features	Clinical features	Prevalence
↓ability to: Relate to others React to change Language development ↓IQ (usually) Ritualistic/stereotyped behaviours	Short attention span Distractability Overactivity Impulsivity	↑in boys 10% age 5, 5% age 10, 1% age 15
Prognosis	Aetiology	Aetiology
Poor Better if: IQ normal Speaking by age of 6	Genetic Dietary Poverty Parental alcohol abuse	Positive FH Unsettling family events Development delay Behaviour problems
Asberger's syndrome	Management	Management
Similar to autism **but** Later onset Normal IQ Schizoid personality Frequent elective mutism	Behaviour modification Exclusion diet Psychostimulants (e.g. methylphenidate)	Exclude physical cause (e.g. UTI) Parental reassurance Behavioural Star chart, pad and bell, imipramine
		Encopresis
		Definition
		Inappropriate deposition of normal stool
		Prevalence
		2% boys, 1% girls at age 8
		Aetiology
		Anger, regression, emotional disturbance (NB sexual abuse) Low IQ
		Management
		Ignore soiling Avoid punishment Star chart
		Prognosis
		90% improve

Developmental disorders

Autism is the most important pervasive developmental disorder (PDD). It is present in about 2/10 000 children with a male/female ratio of 3–4 : 1 and is more common in social classes I and II. Essential features of the disorders are an inability to relate to other people and to changing situations. The onset is before the age of 30 months and can even occur in the first few months (called 'no onset' type). Three features are regarded as essential to the diagnosis: a pervasive failure to make social relationships (aloofness, lack of eye contact, etc.); major defects in language development; and resistance to change with associated ritualistic and/or manneristic behaviours. These may all reflect an inability to process emotional cues. Psychotic phenomena are absent. Affected children often develop inappropriate attachments to unusual objects, have a restricted range of interests and activities, exhibit stereotyped behaviours (rocking, twirling, etc.) and have unpredictable outbursts of screaming or laughter. Although the majority are of limited intelligence (IQ >100 in only 5%), some autistic children have isolated skills (rote memory, computation). Learning disability, deafness and childhood schizophrenia must be considered in the differential diagnosis. Organic factors are strongly implicated in the aetiology: these include genetic loading and perinatal complications. Behavioural treatments, particularly operant conditioning, may reduce stereotypies and encourage more normal development and social functioning. Family support and counselling is crucial. Prognosis is poor with persistent impairments in 60% and further deterioration in 20%; only 15% achieve fully independent functioning. Outcome is considerably better in those in the normal intellectual range and if speech has developed by the age of 6. *Asberger's syndrome* is a less severe form of PDD with later onset, normal intelligence and schizoid personality. Pedantic speech and a preoccupation with obscure facts often occur.

Elective mutism is a marked, emotionally determined selectivity in speaking, such that a child is able to comprehend spoken language, demonstrates language competence in some social situations (most commonly at school), but fails to speak in others. Milder forms of the disorder are common but shortlived (usually at the beginning of schooling), while a clinically significant form is present in 1/1000. Affected children are usually very shy but stubborn and may have had previous speech delay; parents are often overprotective. Recovery occurs in about 50%; those not improving by the age of 10 years usually do badly.

Specific reading retardation (SRR) represents reading difficulties that interfere with academic progress and is not accounted for by low intelligence, poor schooling or visual or auditory difficulties. Prevalence is between 5 and 10% with a marked male and working-class preponderance. Neuropsychological testing often reveals perceptual and/or language deficits and there may be coexistent conduct disorder.

Disorders of elimination

Enuresis refers to non-organic involuntary bladder emptying after the age of 5 years. It can occur by day, by night or both and is defined as secondary if there has been a period of urinary continence and primary if not. Prevalence is 10% at age 5, 5% at age 10 and 1% at age 15 years. Male/female ratio is 2 : 1. Aetiological factors include positive family history, unsettling family events, developmental delay and other behavioural problems in the child. Management involves the exclusion of physical pathology (especially urinary infection), parental reassurance and the institution of a behavioural programme (star chart and/or bell and pad). Tricyclic antidepressants are effective (mechanism unclear), but relapse is frequent when they are discontinued. Anticholinergic drugs (oxybutinin) and synthetic antidiuretic hormone (desmopressin) are increasingly used. Ninety per cent resolve by adolescence.

Encopresis involves the deposition of a normal or near normal stool in inappropriate places in the presence of normal bowel control. Most children are faecally continent by the age of 4 years. Prevalence is about 2% in boys and 1% in girls at age 8 years. Encopresis may reflect anger (with deposits positioned to cause maximum distress) or regression, in children unable to cope with the increasing independence expected of them. Voluntary faecal retention with subsequent overflow is present in some cases. Encopresis is associated with emotional disturbance and other psychiatric disorders (although none is characteristic) and intelligence is usually average or below. There may be underlying parental marital conflicts, punitive potty training and/or sexual abuse. Treatment aims both to restore normal bowel habit and to improve parent/child relationships. Parents should be encouraged to ignore the soiling and in particular not to punish the child. More specific treatments include behaviour modification (e.g. star chart) and family therapy. Drug treatments are of very little use. Ninety per cent improve within 1 year and almost all cases resolve by adolescence. Associated conduct disorder may, however, persist.

Hyperkinetic disorders

The core hyperkinetic syndrome (also called attention-deficit hyperactivity disorder (ADHD)) is characterized by an early onset (usually 3–8 years) of short attention span, distractibility, overactivity, impulsivity, clumsiness and language delay, which lasts longer than 6 months. It is more common in boys (M/F = 3 : 1), may be 'pervasive' (both at home and school) or 'situational' and is often associated with antisocial behaviour. It is less commonly recognized in the UK (<1%) than in the USA (7%), although this probably reflects UK usage of a narrower concept of ADHD. ADHD frequently coexists with conduct disorder, anxiety, depression and SRR. Comorbidity predicts a poorer prognosis. Children with comorbid ADHD and conduct disorder are at particular risk of substance disorders in adolescence; severe forms are often associated with low intelligence, particularly in the context of brain damage (cerebral palsy, epilepsy). Other aetiological factors may include genetic loading, social adversity, parental alcohol abuse, dietary constituents (lead, tartrazine) and exposure to tranquillizers. Treatment approaches include behaviour modification, exclusion diets and (paradoxically) stimulants such as methylphenidate. Tricyclic antidepressants, clonidine, bupropion and antipsychotics are also sometimes used. Hyperactivity usually lessens by adolescence, although learning difficulties often persist and there is an excess of adult antisocial behaviour.

Psychotic disorders

Psychoses of childhood are rare. The most important are the childhood *schizophrenias* which may be acute in onset (carrying a better prognosis) or have a prodrome of apparent developmental delay. As in adolescence and adulthood there is a genetic predisposition and the presentation is with hallucinations, delusions and thought disorder but with a greater preponderance of motility disturbance, particularly catatonia. Antipsychotics are the mainstay of treatment. The *disintegrative psychoses* of childhood are characterized by normal initial development (to age 4 years) and the subsequent onset of a dementia with social, language and motor regression with prominent stereotypies. The aetiology includes infections (especially subacute sclerosing panencephalitis) and neurometabolic disorders. Prognosis is poor. Mania was thought not to occur before adolescence but is now increasingly recognised.

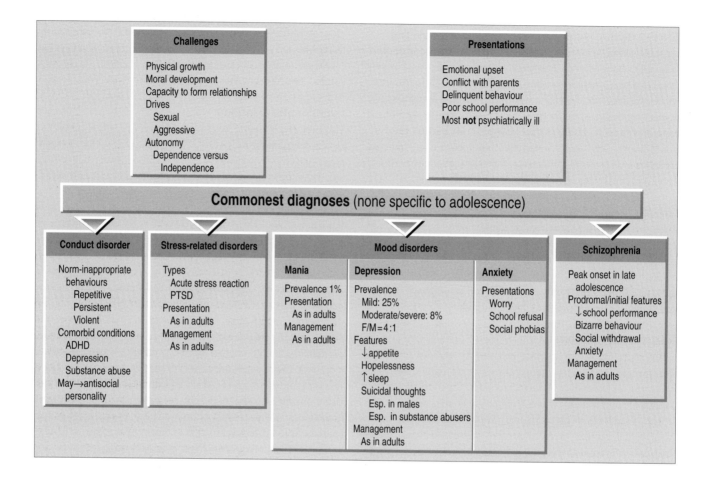

Adolescence stretches from the onset of puberty to the attainment of full physical maturity. It encompasses considerable changes including sudden physical growth, surging sexual and aggressive drives (with associated uncertainties about sexual role, adequacy and identity) and the transition to autonomy and separation from parents (and associated dependence/independence conflict). Moral values may be expected to crystallize and self-esteem grow. Conflicts between individual development and societal expectations may arise, and peer group pressures and influences are crucial. Added challenges include career choice and commitment to work. The capacity for lasting relationships develops in adolescence; difficulties in forming relationships may emerge. Although adolescence is a time of turmoil, true psychiatric disturbance is relatively rare. No psychiatric diagnoses are specific to adolescence; most adult and child psychiatric disorders are seen, often modified by the patient's developmental stage.

Psychiatric assessment in adolescence

Common presentations of psychiatric disorder in adolescence

include emotional upset, conflict with parents, delinquent behaviour and poor school performance. Psychiatric assessment presents a number of challenges. A developmental perspective is crucial, since both level of functioning and apparent 'disorders' must be set against developmental norms. Patients often do not acknowledge their own problems, and referral by parent or school may itself be a source of conflict and distress. Trust and rapport must be built up slowly in the face of resentment, suspicion and the fear of being thought 'mad'. The patient's right to confidentiality must be respected, particularly in the context of sexual abuse. Involving the family is important not only to provide corroborative evidence (the patient's own account often being inadequate or even falsified), but also to build up a picture of the family dynamics that may be crucial in both aetiology and management. A full account of earlier development is particularly important since many adolescent disorders have clear childhood antecedents. Although a number of structured interview schedules and behaviour ratings are available, the diagnostic process is the same as in adults, with most patients having disorders within the DSM or ICD classifications. Comorbidity is, however, even more common than in adults.

Conduct disorder

Conduct disorder (CD) may emerge in adolescence or, if already established, be exacerbated. The essential feature is of conduct violating age-appropriate societal norms. The behaviours are repetitive, persistent and often violent; mugging, theft or even armed robbery are common. CD is associated with low socioeconomic class. 'Solitary' and 'group' patterns of CD are described. Substance abuse (see below), ADHD and depression (see below) often coexist with CD. Coexistent ADHD worsens the prognosis of CD. About one-third of adolescents with CD develop adult antisocial personality disorder, with continuing violent recidivism. Treatment may involve individual and/or family psychotherapy and appropriate management of comorbid conditions. Lithium, haloperidol and carbamazepine may reduce aggressive behaviour. SSRIs may reduce impulsivity, irritability and lability of mood.

Eating disorders

Anorexia nervosa (AN) and bulimia nervosa (BN) are each found in about 1% of adolescents. AN has its peak prevalence in adolescence, and if mild may be difficult to distinguish from age-appropriate preoccupation with dieting. Adolescent onset BN is increasingly common. Obesity is also common in adolescence (prevalence 20–30%). These conditions are discussed in Chapter 11.

Substance abuse

Experimentation with psychoactive substances (tobacco, alcohol, illegal drugs) is common in adolescence, reflecting both adolescent rebellion and the easy availability of the substances. In most cases, there is no lasting harm. Family and social adversity, vulnerable personality, peer pressure and associated CD or depression can contribute to the aetiology of adolescent substance abuse. The hallmarks of problematic abuse are abrupt deterioration in school performance (truancy, low grades, poor discipline), social difficulties (lawbreaking, fights, apparent personality change), slow movements, lethargy, lack of motivation, slurred speech, drowsiness, lack of concentration, absenteeism from school and an unexplained deterioration in physical health. The patient usually denies any problems, and information from school or friends may be vital. There may be other features of CD, and depression is frequent. The rise in adolescent suicide is largely accounted for by substance abusers, and suicide risk must be assessed.

Mood disorders

Mild episodes of depression (characterized by loneliness and low self-esteem) occur in 25% of adolescents and moderate or severe depression in about 8%. Depression is about four times as common in adolescent girls than in boys. Clinical features are essentially the same as in adults, but poor appetite, weight loss and feelings of hopelessness may be more prominent than overt sadness; sleep is more often prolonged than disrupted. Suicidal thoughts (and minor acts of deliberate self-harm) are common; risk of actual suicide (particularly in boys and where there is coexistent substance abuse) must be considered. Anxiety, eating disorders, substance abuse and ADHD all frequently coexist with depression in adolescence. Intervention may include family therapy and individual psychotherapy (particularly cognitive–behaviour; see Chapter 32). Antidepressants (see Chapter 33) are particularly indicated where biological features are prominent.

Mania has a prevalence of up to 1% in adolescence; the presentation and management principles are similar to those in adults. Substance abuse and schizophrenia are the main differential diagnoses.

Anxiety, stress-related disorders

Anxiety most frequently presents as overwhelming, nonspecific worry and repeated demands for reassurance. School refusal (as opposed to truancy) may arise both from specific school-related phobias and from separation anxiety. Social phobias, characterized by avoiding contact with strangers, are also seen. Milder forms may respond to reassurance and advice (to adolescent, parents and school) on coping strategies; in more serious cases, response to relaxation and desensitization is usually favourable. Anxiety may also arise in response to stress, with both acute stress reaction and post-traumatic stress disorder having similar characteristics to their adult counterparts. Management of stress-related anxiety is on similar principles to those used in adults, but the emphasis is more strongly on a behavioural or psychotherapeutic approach, with tranquillizers being resorted to only rarely. SSRIs may be useful in social phobias.

Obsessive–compulsive disorder

Mild obsessionality is common in adolescence; true obsessive–compulsive disorder (OCD) may show prominent obsessional slowness, and behaviour sufficiently bizarre to resemble schizophrenia. Resistance to the thoughts and behaviours may be absent. Tourette's syndrome may coexist. Treatment usually involves both behavioural treatments, e.g. modelling and response prevention, and serotonin-reuptake blocking antidepressants (clomipramine, SSRIs). OCD usually continues into adult life.

Schizophrenia

The peak age of onset of schizophrenia is in late adolescence. Presentation is usually with deteriorating school performance; clinical features are otherwise as in adult life. In younger adolescents, initial presentation is often with bizarre behaviour, social withdrawal and anxiety, with only fleeting first-rank symptoms. The differential diagnosis includes organic states, affective psychosis, drug induced psychosis, adolescent crises and schizoid personality. Antipsychotics (despite frequent sensitivity to sedative and extrapyramidal side-effects) and rehabilitation are the mainstays of management.

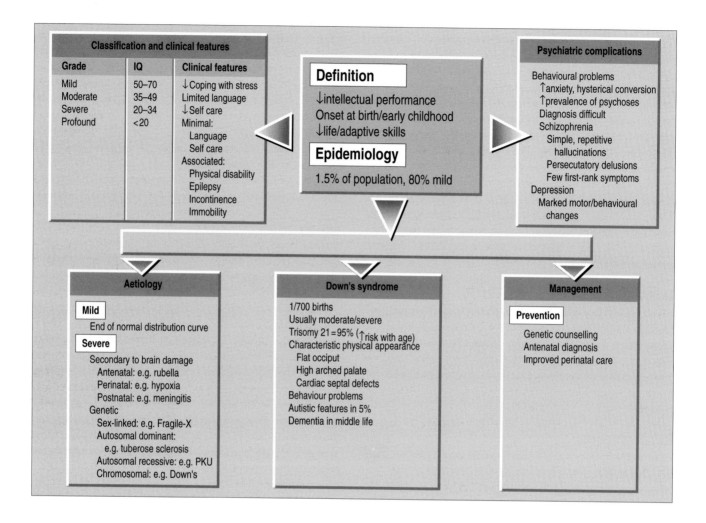

Classification and clinical features

Grade	IQ	Clinical features
Mild	50–70	↓Coping with stress
Moderate	35–49	Limited language
Severe	20–34	↓Self care

Profound	<20	Minimal:
		  Language
		  Self care
		Associated:
		  Physical disability
		  Epilepsy
		  Incontinence
		  Immobility

Definition

↓intellectual performance
Onset at birth/early childhood
↓life/adaptive skills

Epidemiology

1.5% of population, 80% mild

Psychiatric complications

Behavioural problems
  ↑anxiety, hysterical conversion
  ↑prevalence of psychoses
Diagnosis difficult
Schizophrenia
  Simple, repetitive
  hallucinations
  Persecutatory delusions
  Few first-rank symptoms
Depression
  Marked motor/behavioural
  changes

Aetiology

Mild
End of normal distribution curve

Severe
Secondary to brain damage
  Antenatal: e.g. rubella
  Perinatal: e.g. hypoxia
  Postnatal: e.g. meningitis
Genetic
  Sex-linked: e.g. Fragile-X
  Autosomal dominant:
    e.g. tuberose sclerosis
  Autosomal recessive: e.g. PKU
  Chromosomal: e.g. Down's

Down's syndrome

1/700 births
Usually moderate/severe
Trisomy 21 = 95% (↑risk with age)
Characteristic physical appearance
  Flat occiput
  High arched palate
  Cardiac septal defects
Behaviour problems
Autistic features in 5%
Dementia in middle life

Management

Prevention
Genetic counselling
Antenatal diagnosis
Improved perinatal care

Definition

Learning disability (LD; referred to as mental retardation in current classificatory systems) has three main components: low intellectual performance; onset at birth or in early childhood; reduced life/adaptive skills.

Classification and clinical features

LD can be conceptualized in terms of the primary impairment that causes it, the consequent disability and any resultant social handicap (including family difficulties). Intellectual impairment is classified as mild (IQ 50–70); moderate (35–49); severe (20–34) and profound (<20). Mild LD is not usually associated with abnormalities in appearance or behaviour; language, sensory and motor abnormalities are slight or absent. The problem is usually not apparent until school age. Adults with mild LD may have difficulty in coping with stress and often need support with more complex areas of social functioning, such as parenting and handling finance. The majority are, however, able to

live independently in the community and sustain some employment. People with moderate LD usually have limited but useful language. Severe and profound LD are associated with very limited verbal and self-care skills; associated physical handicaps (epilepsy in 33%, incontinence in about 10%, inability to walk in about 15%) are very common. Communication may be facilitated by pointing, tagging or signing. Psychiatric disorder (including behavioural disturbance) has a high prevalence in people with LD but is not integral to it. Behavioural disturbance is increasingly common with increasing severity of LD, occurring in up to 40% of children and 20% of adults with severe LD. This may include purposeless or self-injurious behaviour or inappropriate sexual behaviour such as masturbation in public.

LD is present in about 1.5% of the population. Eighty per cent of cases have mild LD, about 12% moderate and 7% are severely affected. Only 1% are profoundly affected. The prevalence of LD has not fallen despite recent reductions in the incidence of severe LD—this reflects concurrent improvements in prevention (see below) and survival.

Mild LD is not usually associated with specific causes and represents the bottom end of a normal distribution curve for IQ; there is a considerable genetic contribution reflecting the high heritability of IQ in general. The close correlation between low parental and low child IQ is, however, due in part to (potentially reversible) social and educational deprivation. More severe LD is usually related to specific brain damage. Causes may be antenatal (genetic, infective, hypoxic, toxic or related to maternal disease such as toxaemia of pregnancy), perinatal (prematurity, birth hypoxia, intracerebral bleed) or postnatal (infection, injury (particularly non-accidental), malnutrition, hormonal, metabolic, toxic, epileptic). Genetic causes may be chromosomal, e.g. Down's, Klinefelter's and Turner's syndromes, sex-linked (Fragile X, Lesch–Nyhan), autosomal dominant (tuberose sclerosis, neurofibromatosis) and autosomal recessive, the latter usually associated with specific metabolic disorders such as phenylketonuria. Fragile X is the second commonest cause of AD and accounts for 8% of males with LD. It is due to an expansion of a DNA triplet sequence which motivates the FMR-1 gene. Physical signs include large head and ears, connective tissue disorders and mitral valve prolapse. Psychiatric features include abnormal speech, impulsivity and hyperactivity. Four percent have autistic features. The most important antenatal infective agents are toxoplasma, rubella and cytomegalovirus. Perinatal injury frequently causes cerebral palsy (which may be associated with normal intelligence) as well as LD. Autism (see Chapter 22) is usually, although not invariably associated with LD.

Down's syndrome

Down's syndrome (DS) is the commonest specific cause of LD, affecting about 1/700 births. The LD is usually moderate or severe, although only mild LD is present in 15%. Individuals with DS may be stubborn, oppositional and impulsive. Autistic features are present in 5%. In 95% of cases there is trisomy of chromosome 21, risk of which increases with increasing maternal age (1/50 births with maternal age >45). In the remainder, DS is the result of translocation of chromosome 21 material; parents and siblings may be carriers. DS is associated with several physical abnormalities including flat occiput, oblique palpebral fissures, small mouth with high arched palate and broad hands with a single transverse palmar crease. Cardiac septal defects are common and used to result in high early mortality; they are now often corrected. Hypothyroidism is common. Post-mortem studies of people with DS indicate that those surviving beyond the age of 50 years invariably develop neuropathological changes akin to Alzheimer's disease (see Chapter 18); clinical dementia is, however, not always apparent in life.

Psychiatric illness (dual diagnosis)

Challenging behaviours are common in both children and adults with LD and are often related to psychiatric disorder. Making specific psychiatric diagnoses is, however, difficult (particularly in subjects with moderate or severe LD) because of coexisting language deficits. Studies using appropriately structured interviews, detailed behavioural observation and carer data reveal that the prevalence of several psychiatric disorders is increased. Rates are higher in institutional than in community populations. Schizophrenia has a prevalence of 3% and usually presents with simple and repetitive hallucinations and unelaborated, usually persecutory, delusions; these usually lack the complexity of 'first-rank' symptoms (see Chapter 3). The diagnosis of depression rests more on motor and behavioural changes (reduced sleep, retardation, tearfulness, etc.) than verbal expressions of depressed mood; similarly, mania usually presents as overactive and/or irritable behaviour. Phobic anxiety and hysterical conversion symptoms are both common as are psychological reactions to adverse life events. These are, however, often not recognized as such by carers. Genetic, organic (particularly epilepsy), psychological (frustration) and social factors such as family tension, may all contribute to the excess of psychiatric problems associated with LD.

Prevention

Prevention of LD may be attempted before birth through genetic counselling and antenatal diagnosis; in particular, DS may be detected by amniocentesis or chorionic villus sampling, with the option of termination of pregnancy. Improved perinatal care reduces the risk of brain injury, and early detection of hormonal or metabolic problems (myxoedema, phenylketonuria) may allow treatment before LD sets in. There is some evidence that educational intervention in children of mothers with mild LD may enhance their educational performance (although not necessarily their IQ) and reduce risk of conduct disorder.

Management

The movement towards community care has enabled the great majority of people with LD to live in a domestic rather than an institutional setting, usually with their families. Support is provided by the GP and through educational and social services. Educational support for children with mild LD is usually within mainstream schools; in adult life they may need continuing support to hold down open-market jobs. Further training may enable adults with moderate LD to work in appropriate sheltered settings; a small minority (with severe or profound LD and, usually, associated behavioural problems) nonetheless need residential care. Specialist support provided by multidisiplinary community teams involves coordination of local services, assessment of individuals and management of any concurrent mental illness identified, as well as social skills and problem training, and support with finances and accommodation. The latter requires a high index of suspicion and similar treatment principles to those in patients of normal intelligence, with a greater emphasis on behavioural techniques and on working with families/carers.

25 Consultation–liaison psychiatry

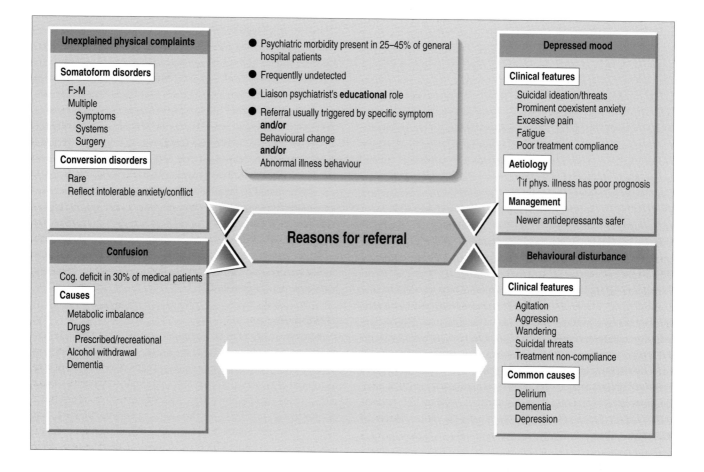

Unexplained physical complaints

Somatoform disorders

F>M
Multiple
  Symptoms
  Systems
  Surgery

Conversion disorders

Rare
Reflect intolerable anxiety/conflict

Confusion

Cog. deficit in 30% of medical patients

Causes

Metabolic imbalance
Drugs
  Prescribed/recreational
Alcohol withdrawal
Dementia

- Psychiatric morbidity present in 25–45% of general hospital patients
- Frequentlly undetected
- Liaison psychiatrist's **educational** role
- Referral usually triggered by specific symptom **and/or** Behavioural change **and/or** Abnormal illness behaviour

Reasons for referral

Depressed mood

Clinical features

Suicidal ideation/threats
Prominent coexistent anxiety
Excessive pain
Fatigue
Poor treatment compliance

Aetiology

↑if phys. illness has poor prognosis

Management

Newer antidepressants safer

Behavioural disturbance

Clinical features

Agitation
Aggression
Wandering
Suicidal threats
Treatment non-compliance

Common causes

Delirium
Dementia
Depression

Consultation–liaison psychiatry refers to the practice of psychiatry on general hospital wards or by the joint care and management of people with both medical and psychological difficulties by physicians and psychiatrists. The narrower and outmoded concept of 'psychosomatic disorders' originally refer to somatic conditions in which there was a structural change or lesion in a target end organ: the aetiology was primarily psychological such as chronic stress and the effects were mediated via the hypothalamic/pituitary axis. Such conditions would include peptic ulceration, asthma, hypertension and certain types of dementia. It is now recognized that psychiatric morbidity (consisting mainly of organic disorders, depression and anxiety) is present in a high (25–45%) proportion of medical and surgical patients, largely irrespective of their primary diagnosis. This reflects both the psychiatric disturbances secondary to physical illness and the increased physical vulnerability that psychiatric difficulties impart. Psychiatric disorder may be important in mediating the established link between adverse life events and physical illness. In addition, abnormalities of personality may predispose to specific physical illness. Aggressiveness, hostility

driving and competitive striving ('type A behaviours') may, for example, predispose to myocardial infarction, and emotional suppression, unassertiveness and overcompliance to cancer.

Rates of referral by physicians and surgeons to the liaison psychiatrist are generally low. Referrals are not always for a specific suspected psychiatric illness. They may be triggered by behavioural disturbance, where real physical symptoms are exaggerated or denied (abnormal illness behaviour), or by failure to find a clear cause for persistent physical symptoms. Underreferral may reflect not only underdetection, but physicians' belief that emotional disorders are simply an understandable response to physical illness, and fear that psychiatric referral will itself generate anxiety or resentment.

The review below will concentrate on principles of managing problems arising in individual medical or surgical patients for whom the liaison psychiatrist may need to provide follow-up as well as acute assessment. The wider brief of liaison psychiatry is educational, in encouraging awareness of psychological aspects of medical illness and thereby enabling earlier detection of individual problems.

Coexistent psychiatric disorders in medical or surgical patients

Organic mental disorder must always be considered in any hospital patient presenting with alteration of behaviour or mood, particularly where there is evidence of cognitive impairment. As many as 30% of acute medical patients have some cognitive deficit, reflecting in part the vulnerability of the aged both to cognitive and physical disorders. Delirium (see Chapter 17) is characterized by impaired attention, clouding of conciousness, fluctuating conciousness, labile affect, disorientation and perceptual disturbance. Common underlying causes in medical patients (usually reversible if identified in time) include metabolic imbalance (reflecting major body system failure), stroke, drugs (both prescribed and recreational) and alcohol withdrawal. Dementia (see Chapter 18) may first become apparent in the setting of acute physical illness, as patients reveal their inability to learn to cope in a novel environment and without family support. Dementia is associated with increased length of hospital stay and its early detection may facilitate appropriate discharge planning.

Depressed mood may trigger psychiatric referral of a medical patient. Such depression often has associated *anxiety symptoms* and may represent an adjustment disorder (see Chapter 8), particularly where the concurrent physical illness has a poor prognosis in terms of chronicity (e.g. diabetes), level of incapacitation or life expectancy. Supportive psychotherapy may be helpful in coming to terms with the consequences of illness. Depressive symptoms may become severe and render patients suicidal or non-compliant with treatment. Antidepressants may be beneficial, but the potential cardiotoxicity of tricyclics (as well as the risk of anticholinergic confusion) is particularly important in this vulnerable group, and newer antidepressants (e.g. SSRIs) may be preferred. Structural brain disease or injury can also cause organic mood disorders, the best known example being the link between stroke (particularly following left anterior infarcts) and depression.

Patients with *pre-existing psychiatric illness* may require urgent medical or surgical management. This is particularly likely in the context of alcohol or substance abuse, with their well-established medical complications, and in patients with established depression or schizophrenia who attempt suicide which may lead to multiple injuries. Such patients will need continued psychiatric management with careful monitoring of their mental state under stressful circumstances. This should also include support and reassurance to medical staff. Particular attention should be paid to possible interactions between psychotropic drugs and any new medical condition or treatment.

Other reasons for psychiatric referral

Psychiatric referral is often triggered by chronic physical complaints for which no organic cause can be found. Rarely, this reflects a *conversion disorder* in which intolerable psychic anxiety or stress is 'converted' into more acceptable and bearable physical symptoms. About which the patient seems relatively unconcerned ('**la belle indifference**'). The key to management is detection of the underlying conflict; this may require hypnosis or abreaction.

More common are the group of *somatoform disorders*. Somatization disorder (sometimes known as Briquet's syndrome) is much commoner in women than in men, and is characterized by complaints involving multiple body systems, starting before the age of 30, and often resulting in multiple operations despite the absence of organic disorder. Related conditions include **hypochondriacal** disorder (non-delusional preoccupation with the possibility of serious illness such as cancer, heart disease or AIDS), **somatoform** autonomic disorder (with predominant autonomic dysfunction such as sweating, palpitations or hyperventillation) and persistent somatoform pain disorder (chronic pain without organic basis).

Management of these conditions involves ensuring that there really is no organic basis, and exploring with the patient (and the family) any 'secondary gain' (such as sympathy or avoidance of family conflict) which might be encouraging symptom maintenance.

Pain may trigger psychiatric referral even without clear evidence of somatoform disorder. Depression may underlie such pain or result from it, particularly if organically caused pain is inadequately treated for fear of causing opiate dependence. Chronic pain may respond to antidepressants (especially SSRIs) even in the absence of clearcut depression, and often at doses too low to be antidepressant. Similar considerations apply to *fatigue*, a feature common to many physical and psychiatric illnesses. In particular, the combination of exhaustion after minimal physical activity, poor concentration and muscle tenderness which constitutes myalgic encephalomyelitis shares many features with depression and may respond to antidepressants.

Psychiatric advice may be requested to deal with *behavioural problems* such as agitation, aggressivity, wandering and noncompliance with treatment. Patients presenting with such behavioural disturbance frequently have delirium (which must be excluded or its underlying cause identified and treated as a matter of urgency) or dementia. Suicidal threats or gestures may also cause considerable anxiety in ward nursing staff who may need advice in both assessment and management of suicide risk (see Chapter 7). Multidisciplinary discussion of behavioural problems can often identify triggers to undesirable behaviour and help ward staff find ways of defusing provocative situations. Appropriate advice may also be needed on the use of tranquillizing drugs and on legal implications of ignoring (or respecting) patients' refusal of treatment.

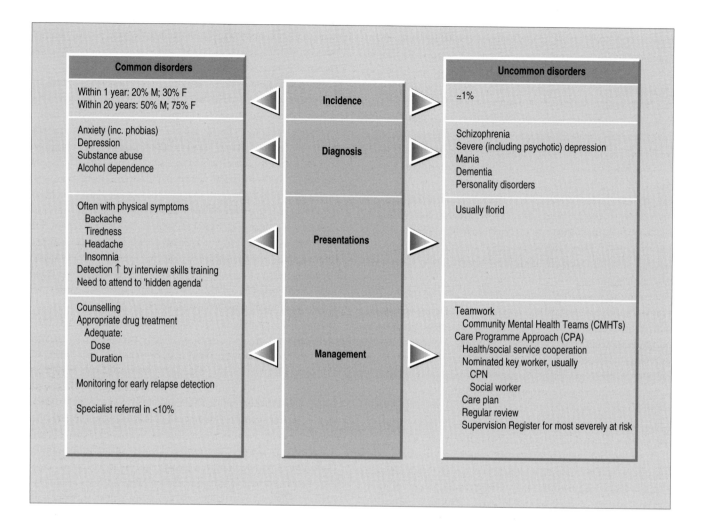

Common disorders		Uncommon disorders
Within 1 year: 20% M; 30% F Within 20 years: 50% M; 75% F	Incidence	≃1%
Anxiety (inc. phobias) Depression Substance abuse Alcohol dependence	Diagnosis	Schizophrenia Severe (including psychotic) depression Mania Dementia Personality disorders

Often with physical symptoms
  Backache
  Tiredness
  Headache
  Insomnia
Detection ↑ by interview skills training
Need to attend to 'hidden agenda'
	Presentations	Usually florid

Counselling
Appropriate drug treatment
  Adequate:
    Dose
    Duration
 	
Monitoring for early relapse detection
 	
Specialist referral in <10%
	Management	Teamwork
		  Community Mental Health Teams (CMHTs)
		Care Programme Approach (CPA)
		  Health/social service cooperation
		  Nominated key worker, usually
		    CPN
		    Social worker
		  Care plan
		  Regular review
		  Supervision Register for most severely at risk

The traditional work of psychiatrists in caring for patients in the hospital in- or out-patient setting accounts for only the tip of the iceberg of significant psychiatric morbidity. Most patients with disabling psychological illness, particularly where this is relatively mild, are dealt with in a primary care setting (if their illness is detected at all). At the other extreme, there has been a considerable shift in locus of care for people with severe and chronic psychiatric illness from the psychiatric hospital into the community. This chapter reviews the delivery of community psychiatric care.

Psychiatry in primary care

Community surveys in the UK and USA suggest that about 25% of the population aged between 18 and 65 years will experience significant psychiatric morbidity within a 1-year period, women outnumbering men by a factor of about 1.5. Over 20 years, the proportion rises to 75% of women and 50% of men. The majority of such illnesses consists of anxiety disorders (including phobias and adjustment reactions) and depression (many patients having features of both). A further important group have substance abuse (including alcohol) problems. A few will have chronic psychotic or personality problems; new psychoses (schizophrenic or affective) are relatively rare. In the elderly, the total prevalence of psychiatric illness is particularly high because of the age-associated rise in prevalence of dementia.

In the UK, virtually the whole population is registered with a general practitioner (GP), and psychiatric morbidity doubles the likelihood of GP consultation. About one-third of patients with significant psychiatric illness will, however, not be recognized by the GP as psychiatrically ill. Patient factors influencing non-detection (which is associated with poor prognosis) include attitude to illness (e.g. not accepting it as psychiatric or as treatable) and to the GP (perceived as not sympathetic or understanding). GP training, attitudes and time available for consultation may also contribute. Detection rates may be increased by interview-skills training, encouraging such factors as eye contact, sensitivity to non-verbal cues and avoidance of exclusive concentration on the presenting complaint at the expense of any 'hidden agenda', of past or chronic problems and of the social and family background. Detection of depression may further be increased by awareness of its frequently somatic presentation (e.g. tiredness, headache, backache, insomnia).

Only about one-eighth of cases detected will be referred to psychiatrists. The decision to refer may reflect the GP's confidence in managing psychiatric illness, the patient's wishes, and the accessibility of the psychiatric service, as well as the severity and duration of the patient's illness.

The challenge of primary care psychiatry is to ensure recognition and optimal care for the submerged iceberg of psychiatric morbidity. Minor anxiety disorders respond to counselling (from practice-based counsellors or psychologists) and depressions to antidepressants or, where available, brief cognitive or problem-solving psychotherapy.

Psychiatrists are increasingly involved in GP surgeries, seeing individual patients, giving management advice and teaching GPs and practice staff (particularly practice nurses) about detection and management of common psychiatric conditions. This might, for example, involve advice on psychological management and on when to refer, as well as encouragement to use drug treatments appropriately. In particular, GPs frequently administer antidepressants at suboptimal doses and for too short a time for acute response to occur or (if patients do recover) to minimize risk of relapse.

Community care of severe psychiatric illness

In the past 40 years, there has been a substantial move away from the hospital as the focus of treatment for severe psychiatric illness. Acute admissions have become fewer and briefer, and continuing care beds have dwindled by more than 50%. Factors involved include the effectiveness of psychotropic drugs, an ideological commitment to the closure of asylum-type psychiatric hospitals and reductions in bed numbers as a cost-cutting exercise.

Closing psychiatric beds is no guarantee of adequate community care. Good community care is usually just as expensive as institutional care, but if adequately resourced can avoid institutionalization and has been shown to achieve high standards both in symptom control and in patient and family satisfaction.

In contrast, poor quality 'cheap' community care can result in gross failure, with increasing numbers of homeless people suffering from severe, untreated and unmonitored mental illness. Good community care should be locally accessible. Psychiatrists and community nurses may work from GP surgeries (see above) or in community mental health centres. Patients unable to live independently may be cared for by family or friends (who may themselves need support). This may not be appropriate since close family contact may increase the risk of schizophrenic relapse (high expressed emotion). Professional support may be provided in group homes (peripatetic supervision) or hostels (resident staff). These are usually run by social service or voluntary organizations. Appropriate employment is difficult to secure, but sheltered work or (in the more severely ill) day care and occupational therapy may be crucial in enabling patients to remain in the community. Risk of relapse must always be considered, with careful monitoring and continued medication (e.g. depot antipsychotics) where appropriate. The CPN has an important role in monitoring patients' clinical state and providing practical support as well as in administering depot injections. Other factors in relapse prevention include avoidance of stress and advice against drug and alcohol abuse.

Detailed care plans, e.g. care programme approach (CPA), should be developed for individual patients; these usually involve cooperation between several services (primarily the health and social services but also housing, GP, family, etc.). This implies considerable negotiation and coordination, with full casenote documentation of agreed care plans. The nomination of a 'key worker' (such as the social worker or nurse) as coordinator of the care package is crucial. A further important element is involvement of the family and of the patient him-/herself. The growth of 'user groups' and of the 'patient advocacy' movement has helped encourage this.

In the UK this approach has been formalized within the 1991 Community Care Act which stipulates that health and social services in particular should agree and monitor care plans for the more severely ill patients. More recently, increasing concern in the UK about the potential risk of self-harm or violence in some severely mentally ill people has led to further legislation requiring that patients at particular risk be placed on a 'supervision register' to ensure adequate monitoring and rapid action if patients fail to comply with treatment.

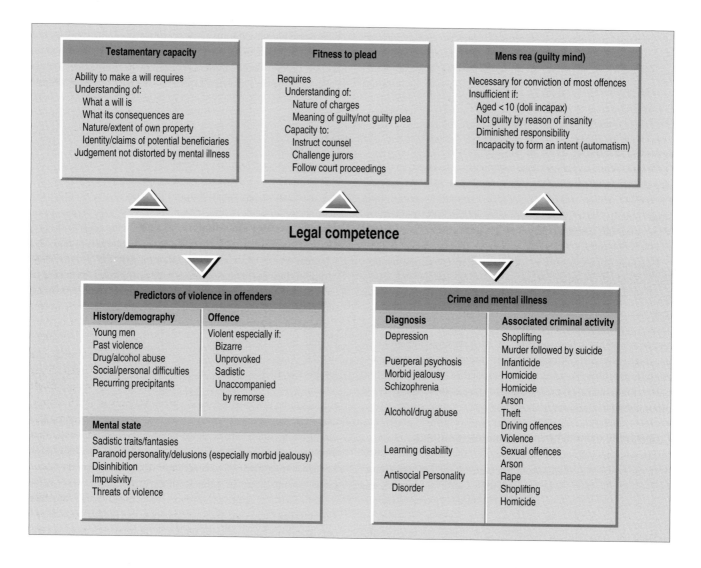

Testamentary capacity
Ability to make a will requires
Understanding of:
What a will is
What its consequences are
Nature/extent of own property
Identity/claims of potential beneficiaries
Judgement not distorted by mental illness

Fitness to plead
Requires
Understanding of:
Nature of charges
Meaning of guilty/not guilty plea
Capacity to:
Instruct counsel
Challenge jurors
Follow court proceedings

Mens rea (guilty mind)
Necessary for conviction of most offences
Insufficient if:
Aged < 10 (doli incapax)
Not guilty by reason of insanity
Diminished responsibility
Incapacity to form an intent (automatism)

Legal competence

Predictors of violence in offenders

History/demography	Offence
Young men	Violent especially if:
Past violence	Bizarre
Drug/alcohol abuse	Unprovoked
Social/personal difficulties	Sadistic
Recurring precipitants	Unaccompanied
	by remorse

Mental state
Sadistic traits/fantasies
Paranoid personality/delusions (especially morbid jealousy)
Disinhibition
Impulsivity
Threats of violence

Crime and mental illness

Diagnosis	Associated criminal activity
Depression	Shoplifting
	Murder followed by suicide
Puerperal psychosis	Infanticide
Morbid jealousy	Homicide
Schizophrenia	Homicide
	Arson
Alcohol/drug abuse	Theft
	Driving offences
	Violence
Learning disability	Sexual offences
	Arson
Antisocial Personality	Rape
Disorder	Shoplifting
	Homicide

Forensic psychiatry concerns the assessment, treatment and rehabilitation of mentally disordered offenders. The main areas covered are links between *crime and mental illness*; the assessment of *legal competence* (to form an intent, to plead, to manage financial affairs or to make a will); the assessment of *dangerousness* (both in offenders and in ordinary psychiatric practice); and mental health legislation (Mental Health Act, see Chapter 28).

Crime and mental illness

Psychiatric illnesses, particularly psychoses and drug- or alcohol-related disorders, are overrepresented in prisoners on remand or serving sentences. This partly reflects a group of urban, homeless, psychiatrically ill, multiple reoffenders; the overall rate of offending by people with a mental illness appears similar to that in the general population. Specific associations

have, however, been demonstrated between offences and psychiatric diagnoses.

Patients with *schizophrenia* often commit minor offences such as shoplifting or damage to property. Violence is rare and usually domestic, in response to poor tolerance of family stress. The specific and much publicized link with homicide is usually in the context of florid psychosis secondary to poor treatment compliance.

Depression may be heralded by a minor 'out-of-character' offence (e.g. shoplifting). Depression-related homicide is rare, usually domestic (typically infanticide), often in response to delusions (e.g. believing that the victim is fatally ill and suffering) and frequently followed by suicide. Offences linked to *mania* (fraud, defaulted debt) usually reflect financial irresponsibility.

Alcohol and substance misuse are associated with theft, robbery, assault and homicide. Acute alcohol intoxication weakens inhibitions against offending ('Dutch courage') and is strongly linked with driving offences. Alcohol is often implicated in **morbid jealousy** (see Chapter 36) which may culminate in spousal homicide.

Dementia is associated with shoplifting (forgetting to pay) and with sexual offences (usually reflecting frontal disinhibition). Similarly, subjects with **learning disability** (see Chapter 24) may commit rape or arson. Violent acts may be committed by younger brain-damaged subjects unable to handle stress or frustration.

The link between crime and **antisocial personality disorder** is somewhat circular, since offending may be integral to the diagnosis, but there are specific associations with recidivism and violent offences.

Legal competence

Most mentally ill people retain responsibility for their actions and the capacity to manage their affairs. There are, however, circumstances where the determination of competence is crucial.

Fitness to plead refers to a defendant's competence to mount a defence against charges and consists of the mental capacity to understand the charge, distinguish between guilty and not guilty pleas, instruct lawyers, follow court evidence and challenge jurors. Unfitness is for a jury to decide. If upheld, a trial of the facts may nonetheless take place, with acquittal if the facts are not established and flexibility of sentence if proven.

For guilt (of most crimes) to be established, it is necessary to demonstrate that the defendant was 'criminally responsible', possessing the **mens rea** (MR) to commit the offence. MR may be absent by virtue of age, psychiatric illness or automatism. Children under 10 years cannot be criminally responsible, and for those aged 10–14 the prosecution must prove MR. Mental disorder is rarely invoked to deny MR; it must be established that the defendant was mentally ill at the time of the offence, resulting in a 'defect of reason', and that consequently he/she could not tell what he/she was doing or know that it was wrong. If successful, the verdict is 'not guilty by reason of insanity'. This theoretically allows some flexibility of sentence, although in practice usually results in hospital detention. 'Automatism' refers to a dissociation between mind and action (e.g. in the context of epilepsy, sleepwalking or concussion).

In the context of murder charges, conviction may be modified (to manslaughter) on grounds of **diminished responsibility** on the basis of specific 'abnormality of mind' substantially impairing mental responsibility.

Mental disorder (particularly dementia) may impair a person's competence to manage his/her (financial) affairs. Such competence involves understanding of one's property and assets, and any obligations thus incurred. A person may (only while still competent) grant to another a 'Power of Attorney' to manage his/her affairs; this automatically becomes invalid if he/she loses the competence. An 'Enduring Power of Attorney', however, remains valid. The Court of Protection (part of the Supreme Court) can appoint a 'receiver' to manage the affairs of someone who has become incompetent to do so.

The related concept of **testamentary capacity** (competence to make a will; TC) must be fulfilled for a will to be valid. It requires a person to understand the act of making a will; to appreciate the extent of his/her property and assets; and to be aware of who might have a reasonable claim on their estate. If the person is mentally ill, TC implies that his/her judgement should not be clouded regarding the will itself. Delusions or hallucinations only impair TC where they are directly relevant to the will (e.g. delusions of poverty).

Predictors of violence in offenders

'Dangerousness' is a judgment based both on the probability of an undesirable act occurring and the gravity of that act. Although most psychiatrically ill people are never dangerous, and most criminally dangerous acts do not take place in the context of mental illness, the assessment of dangerousness is important in all areas of psychiatry when planning aftercare. It is important to distinguish between crimes against property and violence against the person. An assessment of dangerousness is not complete unless all relevant past (psychiatric and criminal) records have been seen. Violent incidents should be accurately documented and should not be omitted from handover or discharge summaries. The time and date of an incident, the factors preceding it, details of the act itself and the immediate consequences should be accurately recorded at the time. The best guide to future behaviour is past behaviour. The more often an individual has been violent in the past, the more likely a further episode becomes. An offender is particularly likely to be dangerous where past violence has been repeated, sudden, unprovoked, bizarre, sadistic and/or unaccompanied by remorse. Predictors within the current circumstances include intoxication, lack of social support and the likelihood that precipitants of past violence will recur. Pointers in the mental state examination include expressed violent intentions or threats, irritability, disinhibition, delusions (usually persecutory, jealous or depressive) with potentially dangerous consequences and reluctance to accept treatment. Dangerousness may warrant compulsory detention or preclude release from such detention. Resource issues should not be allowed to cloud this judgement. More general issues of risk assessment and management are discussed in Chapter 29.

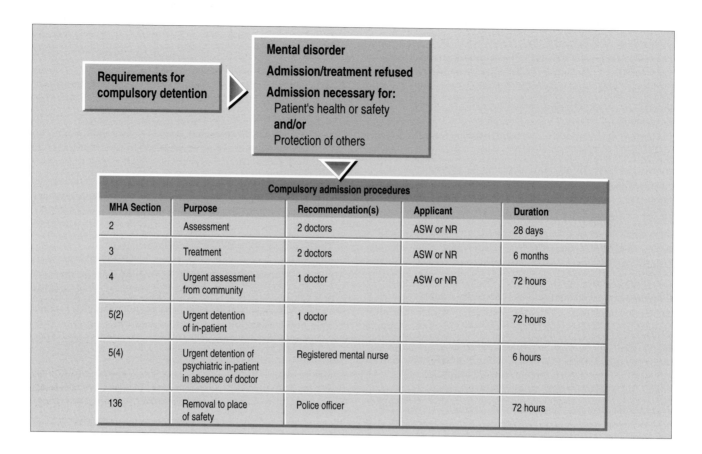

Requirements for compulsory detention

Mental disorder

Admission/treatment refused

Admission necessary for:
Patient's health or safety
and/or
Protection of others

| Compulsory admission procedures | | | | |
MHA Section	Purpose	Recommendation(s)	Applicant	Duration
2	Assessment	2 doctors	ASW or NR	28 days
3	Treatment	2 doctors	ASW or NR	6 months
4	Urgent assessment from community	1 doctor	ASW or NR	72 hours
5(2)	Urgent detention of in-patient	1 doctor		72 hours
5(4)	Urgent detention of psychiatric in-patient in absence of doctor	Registered mental nurse		6 hours
136	Removal to place of safety	Police officer		72 hours

Introduction

The MHA, implemented in England and Wales in 1983, is primarily concerned with the care and treatment of mentally disordered patients. The most important sections address compulsory detention by medical recommendation or court order. The MHA is supervised by the Mental Health Act Commission (MHAC) who have also produced a Code of MHA Practice.

Definitions

The MHA has four categories of mental disorder (MD): mental illness, mental impairment, severe mental impairment (mental retardation) and psychopathic disorder. The MHA does not, however, provide a definition for mental illness. The MHA does not regard promiscuity, immoral conduct, sexual deviancy or dependence on alcohol or drugs as evidence of MD.

General or non-penal compulsory admission procedures

Compulsory admission procedures ('sectioning') may be implemented only if a patient has MD of sufficient severity to warrant detention in hospital in the interests of his/her own health/safety, and/or for the protection/safety of others.

Section 2, admission for assessment (which can include *urgent* treatment) lasts for 28 days. Application is made by a social worker 'approved' under the MHA (ASW) or by the nearest relative (NR) on the basis of recommendations by two medical practitioners, one a specialist 'approved' under the MHA Section 12, and the other preferably with 'previous knowledge' of the patient (usually the GP). Patients may appeal to a Mental Health Review Tribunal (MHRT) within 14 days. MHRTs consist of a lawyer (president), psychiatrist and a lay member (for restricted patients the president is a judge or QC). Patients may be granted legal aid and are able to obtain an independent medical opinion.

Patients may be discharged before the section expires at the discretion of the Responsible Medical Officer (RMO). The MHRT, hospital managers or NR can also implement discharge, although the latter may be barred by the RMO.

Section 3, admission for treatment, lasts 6 months (renewable). The application is by the ASW (after consultation with the NR if possible) or NR. The doctors' recommendation must indicate the nature of the MD, and justify three requirements: (i) the patient suffers from MD warranting treatment in hospital; (ii) for mental impairment or psychopathic disorder that such treatment is likely to alleviate or prevent deterioration; and (iii) that such treatment cannot be provided without detention. The patient or NR may apply to the hospital managers or to a MHRT at any time within the first 6 months and once during each subsequent period of renewal. For treatment to continue beyond the first 3 months, the patient must either consent (and be attested competent to do so by the RMO) or the treatment plan must be agreed necessary by an independent 'second opinion' psychiatrist nominated by the MHAC. Discharge procedures are as for Section 2. *Section 117* requires that a multi-disciplinary meeting be convened to ensure adequate aftercare for any patient discharged from Section 3. *Section 17* requires that patients on Section 2 and 3 can only be placed on leave subject to the RMO's specific instructions.

Section 4, emergency assessment, lasts 72 hours and is applied for by the ASW or NR. One doctor (preferably with previous knowledge of the patient) makes the recommendation on the grounds that admission (otherwise fulfilling Section 2 requirements) is more urgent than Section 2 procedures would allow.

Section 136 empowers a police constable who finds a person in a public place appearing to suffer from an MD to remove him/her to a 'place of safety' for assessment. It is valid for 72 hours.

Section 135, which lasts 72 hours, empowers a police officer or other authorized person acting on a magistrate's warrant to enter premises in order to remove to a place of safety a person who is suffering from an MD, being ill-treated, neglected, not under proper control or is unable to care for themselves (if living alone).

Section 5(2), for patients already in hospital (receiving any form of treatment), is valid for 72 hours, and is on the recommendation of the doctor in charge of the case or his/her nominated deputy. Patients placed on Section 5(2) must subsequently be assessed for Section 2 or 3.

Section 5(4), a nurse's holding power valid for 6 hours, allows urgent detention of a patient already receiving treatment for MD in hospital when a doctor is not able to attend immediately. Only registered mental nurses (RMNs) may make the recommendation; grounds are similar to Section 5(2).

Sections 7 and 8 concern the application for, and description of powers of 'guardianship', intended to ensure that people over 16 years with an MD receive proper care and protection while living in the community. The guardian (who may be a relative) is nominated by the local authority and is empowered to ensure that the individual resides at a specified place, attends specified places and times for treatment, education, training or occupation and allows specified people (e.g. ASWs, doctors) access to their residence.

The Mental Health (Patients in the Community) Act 1995 came into force on April 1 1996. This Act inserts new sections into the existing Mental Health Act 1983. The 1995 Act creates an entirely new legal status of 'After care under supervision (supervised discharge)'. An application for supervised discharge may be made only by the patient's Responsible Medical Officer (RMO) at a time when an individual is detained for treatment under the Mental Health Act 1983 under sections 3, 37, 47 or 48 and is an unrestricted patient. It is meant for people who need to be specifically supervised once they have left hospital to make sure they get the after-care they need. After-care may require the individual to live in a particular place; attend for medical treatment, occupation, education or training at set places and at set times. However, an individual cannot be forced to live at a certain place or take medication or any other kind of treatment without their consent while under supervised discharge. The patient and their nearest relative both have the right to appeal to a Mental Health Review Tribunal (MHRT) when the application for supervised discharge is accepted, and every time it is reviewed.

Penal procedures and orders relating to prisoners

Section 35, empowering a Crown or Magistrates' Court to remand an accused person to a specific hospital for a report, lasts for 28 days, is applied for at trial by defence or prosecution council or by court and requires written or oral evidence from one medical practitioner.

Section 36, empowering a Crown Court to remand an accused individual to hospital for treatment is valid for 28 days and based on two medical reports (one from an 'approved doctor'); the person must be suffering from mental illness or severe mental impairment.

Section 37, empowers a Crown or Magistrates Court to order hospital admission or the reception into guardianship of a person convicted of an imprisonable offence (except murder).

Section 41, a restriction order (by Crown Court only) is based on the oral evidence of one doctor and added to hospital orders. Restricted patients may not be given leave, transferred or discharged, without the consent of the Home Secretary.

Special issues

Section 57 concerns treatment requiring both consent *and* a second opinion (e.g. psychosurgery, surgical implants of hormones).

Section 58 concerns treatment requiring consent *or* a second opinion (e.g. ECT, medications for longer than 6 months).

Legislation for Scotland is different from the rest of the UK.

The Court of Protection is part of the Crown Court and provides for the protection and management of the property and affairs of persons incompetent to do so because of MD.

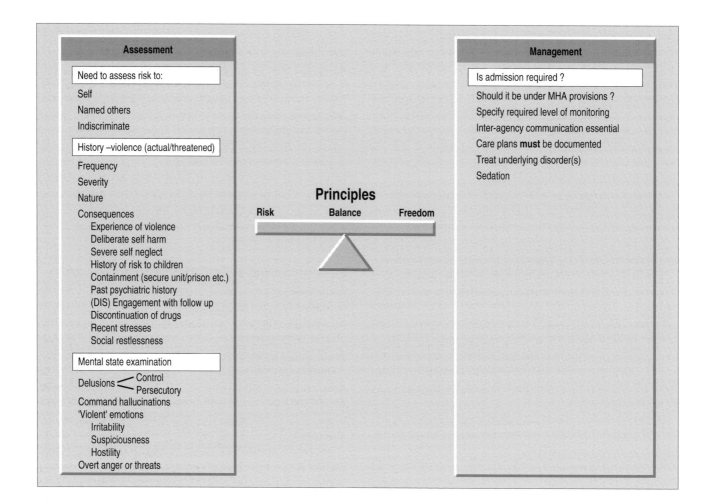

One of the abiding principles in modern psychiatry is that patients' management should be as unrestrictive and normalizing as possible. Inevitably such an approach carries some degree of risk of harm to the patient or to others. There is thus a constant need to balance patients' rights and expectations against the resulting degree of risk. This continuing process, integral both to hospital and community psychiatry, is termed risk assessment and management. Its aim is to reduce risk as far as possible without undue restriction of individual freedoms; risk cannot be eliminated completely. Risks to be considered include those to the self, those specific to named others (e.g. in response to specific persecutory delusions or to a named person in a real or imagined vendetta) and those that are relatively indiscriminate, but are most likely to affect staff and other patients in the immediate vicinity.

Risk assessment

Risk assessment is mandatory when any patient with a psychiatric illness is admitted to hospital; such assessment is also prudent in other contexts such as liaison and general practice psychiatry. Degree of risk is exquisitely sensitive both to changing circumstances and to a patient's changing mental state. Risk assessment should thus be a continuous process of monitoring both the patient and the care setting. The main factors to be considered in assessing the extent to which an individual patient currently poses a risk include aspects of the psychiatric history (including recent risk behaviours) and features within the current mental state.

Psychiatric history

Within the psychiatric history, one must note any history of violence (frequency, severity, nature and most serious harm resulting). A history of exposure to violence or abuse is also important. Any episodes of deliberate self-harm should be documented in detail (circumstances, method, management), as should any evidence of past severe self-neglect. One should also note any history of risk to children. Previous episodes of containment (compulsory detention, treatment in special hospital, secure unit, locked ward, prison or police station) are important and should be noted in detail where possible. Specific additional information within the psychiatric history should include extent of compliance with previous and current psychiatric treatment and aftercare, alcohol or drug misuse (or any other disinhibiting factors), and extent of social integration. Past or current episodes of disengagement from psychiatric follow-up should be noted. Recent stressful life events or changes in life circumstances may be particularly important factors increasing current risk as can recent discontinuation of prescribed or recreational drugs. More generally, evidence of 'social restlessness' such as frequent changes of relationships, work or domicile, indicate increased risk and should be documented.

Most of the above clinical features are indicators of increased risk of harm both to self and to others. Other factors predisposing to deliberate self-harm or actual suicide are discussed in detail in Chapter 7.

Several specific behaviour patterns are associated with increased risk to self or others and should be specifically enquired for in history taking from patient and informant as well as in perusal of case-notes and other documentation. These include episodes of accidental or deliberate harm to self or others, such as overdoses or deliberate self-injury; cigarette-burned bedclothes or deliberate fire-setting; wandering behaviours (particularly in the context of cognitive impairment); and falls consequent on alcohol or drug intoxication. Any such behaviour identified should be documented in detail as to timing, nature and severity of resultant harm.

Acts or threats of violence (to family, strangers, staff or other patients) should also be documented, as should any evidence of sexually inappropriate behaviour. Once again, methods used and resultant injury should be noted. Risk to children should also be assessed and, in this instance in particular, both confidentiality (with regards the patient) and duty to the child must be considered carefully and, if in doubt, advice taken.

Initial assessment

Initial assessment of all patients, particularly those already identified as of high risk, should take place in as safe an environment as possible. The environment in which the patient is being examined or cared for must be assessed and modified to minimise risk. Potential patient access to harmful agents (firearms, knives, other weapons, incendiary devices) should be considered. Where risk is anticipated, one should ensure that senior staff are present where possible. Staff should be trained in 'breakaway' and where possible in 'control and restraint' techniques. Assessment areas should have appropriate alarm facilities and exit routes.

Within the mental state examination (see Chapter 1) key features in risk assessment include persecutory delusions (especially with specific person(s) involved), delusions of control or passivity phenomena, command hallucinations, and emotions with a violent flavour (irritability, suspiciousness, hostility). Overt anger or explicit threats are particularly informative.

At the end of the initial assessment, it should be possible to estimate the level of risk in terms of seriousness, specificity, immediacy and potential for rapid change. This should form the basis of a management plan aimed at risk reduction.

Management

Clinical management of risk involves decisions as to whether admission is necessary, and if so whether such admission should be under the provisions of the Mental Health Act (see Chapter 28) and/or to a psychiatric intensive care unit (PICU) or secure unit. Level of monitoring should be specified both for patients in the community and those in hospital. Medication may play an important role both in treating any underlying psychiatric disorder and also (in patients with high levels of arousal), in inducing sedation or tranquillization (see Chapters 33 and 34). Communication between agencies (particularly Health and Social Services) is crucial in planning future care in the community of patients at high risk who are likely to need considerable supervision that is both practical and acceptable. Care plans and their implementation must be negotiated by all involved parties (including patients themselves and their family and other informal carers), and fully documented.

30 Psychosexual disorders

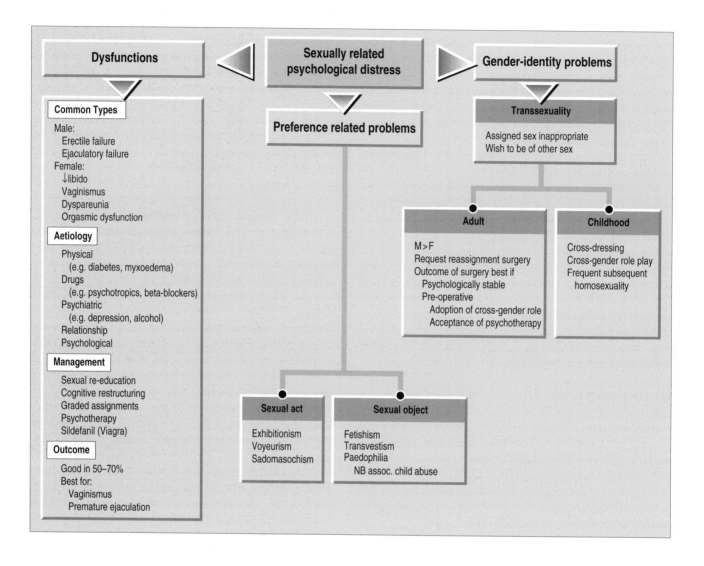

The range of sexual behaviour is extremely wide, with concepts of normality socially or legally, rather than physiologically, determined. Increasing awareness of the potential hazards of sexual freedom (particularly HIV infection), and of what might be expected from a sexual relationship, have encouraged the increasing 'medicalization' of sexuality. Current psychiatric classifications (DSM-IV, ICD-10) emphasize that sexual disorders have an element of psychological distress rather than being defined by behaviour alone. They can conveniently be divided into disorders of sexual *function, preference* and *identity*.

Sexual dysfunctions

Some degree of sexual dissatisfaction is present in as many as 20% of women and 30% of men. The commonest problems identified in both surveys and referrals to sexual disorder clinics are failure of erection and/or ejaculation in men; and low sexual interest, inability to allow penetration (vaginismus), pain on intercourse (dyspareunia), lack of sexual enjoyment and orgasmic dysfunction in women.

Assessment involves detailed history taking from, and examination of, both partners in order to identify the nature of the problem, its time course, the couple's knowledge of and attitudes to sex and the reasons why help is now being sought. Aetiological factors to be considered in the initial assessment include psychological factors, recent life events, specific medical and psychiatric conditions (and their treatment), past sexual abuse and poor general relationship with the sexual partner. Physical conditions impeding sexual function include neurological conditions (e.g. multiple sclerosis), diabetes, myxoedema and pelvic surgery. Sexual dysfunction may be induced by several drugs including beta-blockers, diuretics, antipsychotics (particularly thioridazine), benzodiazepines and tricyclics. Sexual function is often impaired in depression (where loss of libido may reflect generalized anhedonia), alcohol dependence or abuse, and anxiety states, and may be a manifestation of poor psychological adjustment to surgery (particularly mastectomy, colostomy or amputation).

Management increasingly involves a combination of medical and counselling interventions, including treatment of underlying medical or psychiatric conditions and marital therapy. Erectile dysfunction in men is increasingly being treated by physical means such as intracavernosal Caverject, mechanical devices (vacuum pumps, penile bands), oral yohimbine or (rarely) surgical implants. Oral sildefanil (Viagra) has recently been introduced as a treatment for erectile dysfunction. Psychological treatments are essentially cognitive–behavioural, aiming at facilitating communication, decreasing anxiety about performance failure and identifying and exploring underlying psychodynamic problems as well as sexual re-education. This may include traditional sex therapy which (irrespective of the presenting dysfunction) involves the setting of a hierarchy of sexual 'assignments', structured on behavioural principles. Outcome is good in 50–70% of cases, the best results being for premature ejaculation in men and vaginismus in women. Other favourable prognostic factors include good quality of general relationship, high motivation and early progress within treatment.

Disorders of sexual preference (paraphilias)

The paraphilias may be classified into those where the primary deviation is in the focus for the sufferer's initial sexual arousal (rather than the subsequent sexual act), and those where it lies in the nature of the preferred sexual act itself.

It should be noted in this context that homosexuality is not considered a disorder of sexual preference. Subjects who are dissatisfied with their sexual orientation are almost always so because of prejudice or discrimination.

Variations of the sexual object include *paedophilia* (sexual activity or fantasy involving children); *fetishism* (where the object of sexual arousal is an inanimate object (e.g. an item of clothing or a non-genital body part); *transvestism* (where sexual arousal is obtained by cross-dressing); and, more rarely, *bestiality* (sexual activity with animals) and *necrophilia* (intercourse with a dead body). Paedophilia is particularly important because of its link with child pornography and abuse (see Chapter 21).

The aetiology of these conditions is unclear; management usually involves behaviour therapy (which may involve elements both of aversion and of conditioning more appropriate responses). Antiandrogens are sometimes used in paedophilia.

Variations of the sexual act involve the induction of both sexual arousal and (usually) orgasm, by specific actions. Almost all people presenting to the courts or for psychiatric treatment with such variations are men. The commonest form is *exhibitionism* (indecent exposure) in which genital exposure is accompanied by emotional tension and excitement as well as sexual arousal. Exhibitionists make up one-quarter of the sexual offences dealt with by the courts, with psychiatric referral usually by this route. Exhibitionists fall into two main groups: those with aggressive personality traits or even antisocial personality disorders (see Chapter 12) and in whom the act frequently involves masturbation; and those of inhibited temperament, where the exposed penis is often flaccid. Treatment may include psychodynamic, behavioural and hormonal (antiandrogen) components.

Other relatively common variations of the sexual act include *voyeurism* (observing sexual acts), *frotteurism* (rubbing the genitalia against a stranger in a crowded place) and *sadomasochism* (inflicting pain on others (sadism) or having it inflicted on oneself (masochism)). There are no systematic trials of treatment, although behavioural techniques are often used.

Gender identity disorder (GID)

This involves a strong wish to be of the other sex, and a conviction that one's assigned sex is inappropriate. It may occur in children, in whom it is characterized by cross-dressing, taking cross-gender roles in games and fantasy and an attraction for pastimes appropriate to the other gender's stereotype. Boys with GID frequently develop homosexual orientation as adults.

The cardinal feature of GID in adults *(transsexuality)* is a clear wish to live as a member of the other sex, with cross-dressing reflecting this rather than for sexual excitement. Most adult transsexuals are male. Transsexuals usually seek gender-reassignment surgery (with associated hormonal treatment). Outcome following such treatment is best where the patient is otherwise psychologically stable, has adopted the cross-gender role consistently prior to surgery, accepts that surgical treatment is not a 'cure', and is willing to participate in presurgical psychotherapy.

31 Psychiatric aspects of HIV and AIDS

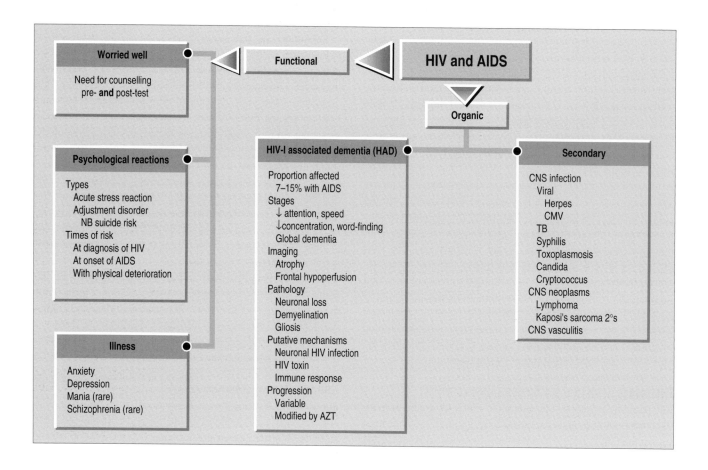

The World Health Organization estimated that at the end of 1998, 33.4 million people were living with HIV or AIDS and a further 13.9 million had died of AIDS–related illnesses. In the developed world the majority of cases are in homosexual men and in intravenous drug abusers, but the incidence of heterosexually spread HIV infection is rising rapidly, particularly in adolescents and in women. Associated psychological problems range from fear of infection in the 'worried well', through psychological reactions to being HIV infected or developing features of AIDS, to functional psychiatric disorders in those with established HIV or full-blown AIDS and neuropsychiatric syndromes resulting both from HIV itself, and from its complications and treatment.

The worried well

People at risk of HIV may become preoccupied with the possibility of becoming infected; this may present with repeated requests for HIV serological testing. HIV testing should never be undertaken without clarification of why the test is being sought, estimation of likelihood of a positive result and advice as to further action whatever the test result. It also provides an opportun-

ity for education on minimizing high-risk behaviour. A request for testing may reflect underlying depression or anxiety which should be excluded or treated as part of the initial assessment. More rarely, patients with psychotic depression or schizophrenia may present with the delusion that they are HIV positive.

Psychological reactions to HIV infection

Patients with HIV may undergo periods of crisis on first learning that they are infected, when they first develop an HIV-related illness or full-blown AIDS and as physical deterioration becomes inexorable. They may react to these crises with acute stress reactions or more insidious adjustment reactions (see Chapter 8). Risk of deliberate self-harm must be considered. This is particularly important in the context of disclosure of a positive HIV-test. Such disclosure should be prearranged and in person; where possible a close friend or family member should be present, and one or more follow-up appointments may be needed. Patients may initially display shock or disavowal; they should be encouraged to ventilate their feelings and supported through the anger and despair that often precede acceptance of the diagnosis. Self-help groups can play an important role.

Functional psychiatric disorders

Depressive symptoms are common at all stages of HIV and AIDS. The diagnosis of depressive illness may be difficult. Low mood may be an understandable reaction to the diagnosis or to progressive disability, and apathy due to organic CNS disease. Anhedonia, hopelessness and suicidal thinking are, however, likely to reflect true depressive illness and warrant treatment. HIV-positive patients may also present with acute mania or schizophrenia-like psychoses. Anxiety is also common, and may respond to behavioural and/or pharmacological treatment. Organic aetiology should be excluded or treated; the principles of management of functional psychoses are not altered by comorbidity with HIV or AIDS.

People with AIDS are often very sensitive to the side-effects of psychotropic drugs. The anticholinergic effects of tricyclic antidepressants can aggravate cognitive deficits, and SSRIs may be preferred. Similarly, benzodiazepines and antipsychotics may also aggravate organic presentations. Choice of psychotropic is often dictated by the patient's physical problems. For example, where depression coexists with the chronic diarrhoea common in AIDS, patients may benefit from the anticholinergic effects of tricyclics but be intolerant of SSRIs.

HIV-induced neuropsychiatric dysfunction

Some subjects infected with HIV (estimates vary between 10 and 90%) develop a self-limiting aseptic meningitis which probably represents the entry of the virus into the CNS. The clinical presentation is usually of a glandular fever-like illness accompanied by neck stiffness, but there may also be a transient confusional state.

Later in the disease, HIV-positive subjects may develop persistent and progressive cognitive changes. These are thought to be a direct manifestation of HIV infection within the brain and are known as HIV-I associated dementia (HAD). HAD develops rarely in patients with AIDS-related complex, and in about 7–15% of those with untreated AIDS.

The early stages of HAD may be apparent only on detailed neuropsychological testing, particularly on measures of psychomotor speed or of sustained attention. Rarely, however, there may be a more acute presentation with a mania-like agitated psychosis accompanied by acute impairment of memory and orientation.

As HAD develops, the picture is of a subcortical dementia in which difficulties become apparent in concentration, word-finding, memory and information processing. The cognitive changes may be accompanied by apathy, social withdrawal and motor dysfunction (hand tremor, deteriorating handwriting,

poor balance). The later stages of HAD are characterized by a clinical picture similar to that of other dementias, with progressive impairment of daily living skills leading to inability to converse and full physical dependency.

Structural imaging scans in HAD reveal cortical atrophy (which may precede cognitive impairments) and, less frequently, patchy areas of low attenuation in the white matter. Single photo emission tomography (SPECT) studies reveal frontal hypoperfusion. The main pathological abnormalities are demyelination and gliosis, more marked in white matter, and grey-matter neuronal loss. Postulated pathogenic mechanisms include direct infection of neurons and glia by HIV, toxin production and host immune responses.

The prognosis of HAD is variable and treatment dependent. Before azidothymidine (AZT) came into routine use in the treatment of AIDS, some patients with HAD showed very rapid cognitive deterioration over weeks. AZT may temporarily reverse or delay progression of the cognitive deficits of early HAD, and subsequent cognitive decline can take 1 year or more. There is early evidence that newer combination antiviral therapies can slow or reverse HAD, though their efficiencies vary. It is possible that in the future combination therapies, immune stimulation and/or selective vaccines may prevent HAD. There are currently no other specific treatments for HAD. Agitation may require antipsychotics, although HAD renders patients particularly vulnerable to severe and prolonged extrapyramidal side-effects. Psychostimulants such as methylphenidate may transiently improve both mood and cognitive performance.

Neuropsychiatric manifestations of complications of HIV

Severely immunocompromised AIDS patients are vulnerable to a variety of opportunistic CNS infections. Viral infections include herpes and cytomegalovirus. Non-viral infections are also common. These include tuberculosis, syphilis, toxoplasmosis, candidiasis and cryptococcal meningitis. AIDS also renders patients vulnerable to CNS neoplasia, particularly lymphoma (primary or secondary) and metastatic Kaposi's sarcoma. CNS vasculitis can result in haemorrhage or infarction. These complications may present with non-specific cognitive deterioration or more florid acute confusional states, with or without focal neurological signs.

Treatments directed at HIV and its complications can also result in neuropsychiatric syndromes. AZT can cause drowsiness or, rarely, a mania-like syndrome. Pentamidine (used in the treatment and prophylaxis of cryptococcal lung infections) may induce hypoglycaemia and resultant confusion.

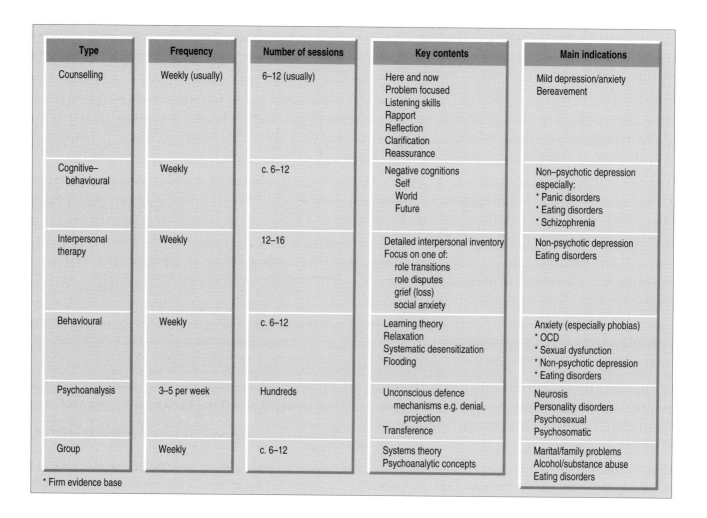

Type	Frequency	Number of sessions	Key contents	Main indications
Counselling	Weekly (usually)	6–12 (usually)	Here and now Problem focused Listening skills Rapport Reflection Clarification Reassurance	Mild depression/anxiety Bereavement

Cognitive–behavioural	Weekly	c. 6–12	Negative cognitions
			  Self
			  World
			  Future
				Non–psychotic depression
				especially:
				* Panic disorders
				* Eating disorders
				* Schizophrenia

Interpersonal therapy	Weekly	12–16	Detailed interpersonal inventory
			Focus on one of:
			  role transitions
			  role disputes
			  grief (loss)
			  social anxiety
				Non-psychotic depression
				Eating disorders

Behavioural	Weekly	c. 6–12	Learning theory Relaxation Systematic desensitization Flooding	Anxiety (especially phobias) * OCD * Sexual dysfunction * Non-psychotic depression * Eating disorders

Psychoanalysis	3–5 per week	Hundreds	Unconscious defence
			  mechanisms e.g. denial,
			    projection
			Transference
				Neurosis
				Personality disorders
				Psychosexual
				Psychosomatic

Group	Weekly	c. 6–12	Systems theory Psychoanalytic concepts	Marital/family problems Alcohol/substance abuse Eating disorders

* Firm evidence base

Psychotherapy (based on verbal communication between client/patient (CP) and doctor, and the relationship between them) aims to help individual CPs cope, adjust to life, relieve uncomfortable psychological symptoms, improve their mental state and/or foster their rehabilitation, enabling them to lead as full a life as possible.

Counselling

The term counselling covers a wide range of different and largely unproven interventions. The most widely practiced is Person Centred Counselling. This is non-directive; the aim is to 'be with' the CP in a meaningful way. Empathy, unconditional positivity and genuineness are seen as the main therapeutic ingredients. Other types of counselling involving provision of information, problem solving and support have been shown to be effective in primary care and general medical settings.

Supportive psychotherapy

Supportive psychotherapy, the simplest form of psychotherapy, assesses the CP's life situation by allowing the CP to talk freely about his-/herself, symptoms and problems. The therapist then facilitates changes, enabling the CP to be more functional, with decreased anxiety and restoration or maintenance of the status quo. CPs are seen weekly for several weeks or months. Brief (one to three sessions) crisis intervention helps support an individual at times of stress or crisis and prevent breakdown of functioning. The therapist works with the CP's symptoms rather than unconscious processes, and does not aim at major personality changes or giving insight. He/she listens to the CP, understands the problems and reinforces psychological defence mechanisms. Cooperation from the CP (trying to solve problems, rather than dependence and regression) is stressed. Suggested steps are establishing rapport, facilitating the expression of affect/emotions (e.g. grief, anger), followed by reflection, clarification, reassurance from the therapist, facilitation of the CP's understanding of his/her own feelings and encouragement of problem-solving behaviour.

Psychoanalysis

Psychoanalysis, a form of psychotherapy, also refers to the school of psychology founded by Sigmund Freud. It stresses the importance of childhood experience in forming the personality. Classical Freudian theory has been modified by his followers, but the central notion remains that human behaviour is determined predominantly by unconscious forces derived from primitive emotional needs, rather than by reason. The analyst aims to resolve long-standing underlying conflicts (and unconscious defence mechanisms such as denial and repression), to promote personal growth, and to modify the personality of the CP by intensive exploration of the unconscious using free-association (allowing the CP to say aloud whatever enters his/her mind) and interpretation. An analyst sees a CP four or five times a week for 50–60 minutes for 2–5 years. One of the key therapeutic tools is the transference (the process by which the patient transfers to the analyst strong emotions experienced in relation to early important relationships). The related concept of counter-transference refers to the thoughts and feelings the analyst experiences in response to the CP.

Brief psychodynamic psychotherapy

Brief Psychodynamic Psychotherapy (BPP), is related to but more widely available than psychoanalysis. It also aims to facilitate changes by detecting and resolving underlying psychological conflicts which cause interpersonal problems. Treatment sessions are less frequent (one to two times a week) and the CP and therapist face each other.

Interpersonal psychotherapy

Interpersonal therapy (IPT) was devised in the late 1960s by Weissman and Klerman and arises from research linking interpersonal relationships, life events and social networks with depression (see Chapter 5). IPT was, initially, used specifically in the treatment of non-psychotic depressive disorders. A detailed interpersonal inventory is taken of all close relationships. A particular focus is chosen such as a role transition (e.g. promotion, loss of job, becoming a parent) or a role dispute within an important relationship. Other possible foci are grief (loss) and social anxiety/ineffectiveness. Fluctuations in the area of focus are carefully matched to fluctuating symptoms of depression on the basis that if the interpersonal difficulty can be helped the depression will be alleviated. IPT has been used successfully in eating disorders.

Cognitive–behaviour therapy

Cognitive–Behaviour Therapy (CBT) was initially devised by Beck for treating depressive illness. It was based on observations that depressed patients entertain negatively biased cognitions (thoughts) of themselves, their future and the environment/world (Beck's cognitive triad). These cognitive distortions ('silent assumptions') are thought to arise from early traumatic experiences, and, in depression, are manifest as depressive cognitions ('automatic thoughts') which the CP is encouraged to challenge. CBT, employing directive methods and dealing with current problems, seeks to change these important inner attitudes. CBT is now also used in the treatment of generalized and phobic anxiety, eating disorders (particularly bulimia), schizophrenia and some personality disorders.

Behaviour therapy

Behaviour Therapy (BT), based on learning theory, concentrates on changing behaviour and is directive. Specific techniques include exposure, response prevention, habituation and thought stopping. Operant conditioning techniques involve encouraging desirable behaviours by positive reinforcement, and discouraging undesirable behaviours by withholding reinforcement (extinction). In aversion therapy, the CP is given an unpleasant stimulus (e.g. electric shock) when behaviour is undesirable. During flooding, the CP is rapidly exposed to an anxiety-producing stimulus or imagination thereof. In systematic desensitization (SD) the CP experiences graded exposure to a hierarchy of increasing anxiety producing situations/objects. Reciprocal inhibition couples SD with a response incompatible with anxiety, such as relaxation or eating.

More recently, BT has shifted towards using activity schedules, planning, reducing avoidance and self-monitoring, backed by education and information. Such regimes are effective in a wide range of disorders including depression, recovery after coma or myocardial infarction and pain management.

Eye movement desensitization and reprocessing

Eye Movement Desensitization and Reprocessing (EMDR) combines a specific attentional task (tracking a rapidly moving object by eye) with a cognitive one (holding images and feelings of trauma in the mind). EMDR has been shown to be rapidly effective in Post Traumatic Stress Disorder (see Chapter 8).

Group therapy, in this the emphasis is on the interrelationships within the group where problems are shared. Groups (small—12 members are ideal) meet weekly, and run for months to years. The therapist (who sits in the group) adopts a non-directive role but discourages CPs from avoiding 'psychological work' (e.g. by remaining silent or talking about irrelevancies).

Family systems therapy, has a central premise that problems have arisen with the system of family functioning rather than just in the individual. The expectation is that improved family functioning will result in the improvement of the index 'case'.

Milieu therapy, within an in-patient 'Therapeutic Community', employs all residents (CPs) and staff to give support to individual CPs, promoting more adaptive coping skills and modification of behaviour by peer pressure.

Transactional analysis (TA) was founded by Eric Berne who noted that individuals related to each other in different ego states (children, adults, parents). In TA these ego states are explored/interpreted to the CP (individually or in groups), aiming at eventual predominantly adult functioning.

33 Physical treatments I

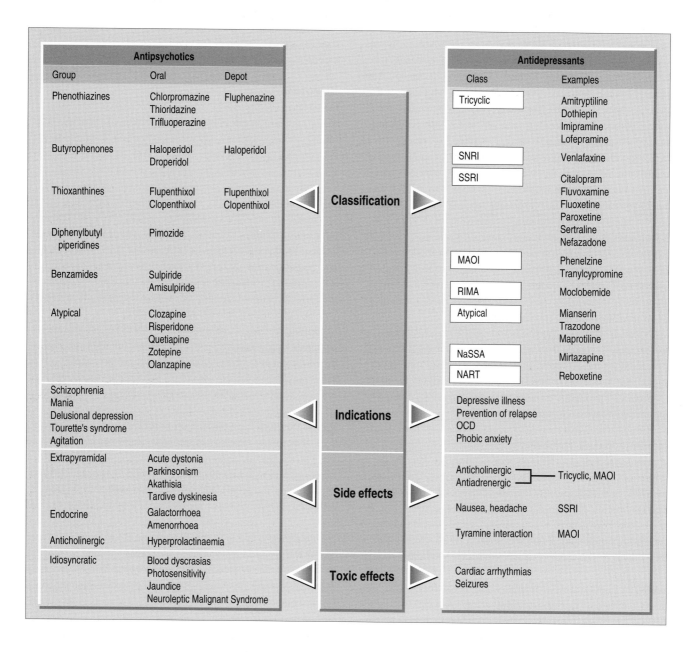

Antipsychotics		
Group	**Oral**	**Depot**
Phenothiazines	Chlorpromazine Thioridazine Trifluoperazine	Fluphenazine
Butyrophenones	Haloperidol Droperidol	Haloperidol
Thioxanthines	Flupenthixol Clopenthixol	Flupenthixol Clopenthixol
Diphenylbutyl piperidines	Pimozide	
Benzamides	Sulpiride Amisulpiride	
Atypical	Clozapine Risperidone Quetiapine Zotepine Olanzapine	
Schizophrenia Mania Delusional depression Tourette's syndrome Agitation		
Extrapyramidal	Acute dystonia Parkinsonism Akathisia Tardive dyskinesia	
Endocrine	Galactorrhoea Amenorrhoea	
Anticholinergic	Hyperprolactinaemia	
Idiosyncratic	Blood dyscrasias Photosensitivity Jaundice Neuroleptic Malignant Syndrome	

Classification / Indications / Side effects / Toxic effects

Antidepressants	
Class	**Examples**
Tricyclic	Amitryptiline Dothiepin Imipramine Lofepramine
SNRI	Venlafaxine
SSRI	Citalopram Fluvoxamine Fluoxetine Paroxetine Sertraline Nefazadone
MAOI	Phenelzine Tranylcypromine
RIMA	Moclobemide
Atypical	Mianserin Trazodone Maprotiline
NaSSA	Mirtazapine
NART	Reboxetine
Depressive illness Prevention of relapse OCD Phobic anxiety	
Anticholinergic Antiadrenergic	Tricyclic, MAOI
Nausea, headache	SSRI
Tyramine interaction	MAOI
Cardiac arrhythmias Seizures	

Physical treatments should always be seen as part of individual patients' management programmes rather than as complete in themselves. There is also no intrinsic antagonism between physical and more social or psychological treatment approaches; indeed, they are usually complementary.

Antipsychotics

These are also known as neuroleptics. The first of them, chlorpromazine, was introduced in 1951 for use in anaesthetic premedication since it induced a state of 'relaxed alertness'. It was soon tried in schizophrenia and noted to reduce delusions and hallucinations without causing excessive sedation.

Drugs currently in use are the phenothiazines (such as chlorpromazine, thioridazine, fluphenazine and trifluoperazine); the butyrophenones (haloperidol, droperidol); the thioxanthenes (flupenthixol, *cis*-clopenthixol); the diphenylbutylpiperidines (pimozide) and the substituted benzamides (sulpiride); and the atypical antipsychotics zotepine, clozapine, olanzapine, quetapine and risperidone.

Mechanism of action. All antipsychotics are potent dopamine-receptor blockers but also block cholinergic, adrenergic and histaminic receptors. Older drugs (phenothiazines and butyrophenones) are relatively non-selective, whereas the benzamides are highly selective blockers of D2 dopamine receptors. The 'atypical' antipsychotics block $5HT_2$ receptors as well as dopamine receptors. Some atypicals block limbic dopamine receptors preferentially to those in the striatum.

Mode of administration. This is usually by mouth, with extensive 'first-pass' metabolism in the liver. Many can also be given by short-acting intramuscular (IM) or intravenous (IV) injection. Some (such as haloperidol and flupenthixol) can be given as esters dissolved in vegetable oil by deep 'depot' IM injection every 1–4 weeks. This bypasses first-pass metabolism and may improve compliance. Depot medication is easier to monitor. The supervising CPN can also act as 'key worker'.

Indications. Antipsychotics are drugs of first choice in the treatment of schizophrenia; they are most effective in alleviating 'positive' symptoms such as delusions, hallucinations, disorders of possession of thought and formal thought disorder; they are also effective in preventing relapse. Clozapine and risperidone may be more effective against 'negative' features (lack of volition and poverty of thought and affect) than other neuroleptics. Major tranquillizers are also effective in the treatment of mania, of Tourette's syndrome and for violent or agitated behaviour in the context of acute confusional states and dementia. They are also used, in combination with antidepressants, in delusional depression.

Side-effects. The most important of these are the extrapyramidal movement disorders. Patients may experience acute dystonic reactions (torticollis, oculogyric crisis, increased muscle tone), parkinsonism or akathisia (psychomotor restlessness). Acute dystonia and parkinsonism reflect drug-induced dopamine/acetylchoine imbalance and respond to anticholinergic drugs such as procyclidine. Akathisia is less responsive to anticholinergics than parkinsonism. Beta-blockers or benzodiazepines may be helpful. Long-term antipsychotics may cause tardive dyskinesia (TD), thought to be due to dopamine-receptor supersensitivity and characterized by abnormal buccolingual masticatory movements and, in severe cases, choreiform trunk and limb movements. Tetrabenazine may reduce the movements of TD as may reduction or cessation of antipsychotics. TD is, however, irreversible in 50% of cases. Weight gain is an important and distressing side effect associated with chronic antipsychotic administration and may adversely effect compliance. Most other side-effects relate to other receptor blockade. Anticholinergic effects include dry mouth, confusion and urinary retention. Postural hypotension and impotence are antiadrenergic effects and sedation probably reflects histamine blockade. Endocrine effects (secondary to dopamine blockade) include hyperprolactinaemia, amenorrhoea and galactorrhoea. Phenothiazines may cause an allergic cholestatic jaundice. Clozapine may cause potentially fatal agranulocytosis and seizures. Despite these risks and the need for regular haematological monitoring, clozapine is increasingly seen as useful in patients unresponsive to or intolerant of standard antipsychotics.

Toxic effects include the neuroleptic malignant syndrome (hyperpyrexia, autonomic instability, confusion and increased muscle tone); and (with phenothiazines) blood dyscrasias, retinal pigmentation, photosensitivity and cholestatic jaundice.

Antidepressants

Drugs currently in use may be divided into the tricyclics (such as imipramine, amitriptyline, dothiepin and lofepramine); the MAOIs such as phenelzine and tranylcypromine and the new reversible inhibitor of MAO-A, or 'RIMA' moclobemide; the SSRIs (citalopram, fluvoxamine, fluoxetine, sertraline and paroxetine); venlafaxine (similar to SSRIs but with some noradrenaline reuptake blockade at high dose and therefore classed as a selective serotonin and noradrenaline reuptake inhibitor (SNRI)); mirtazapine, which has a 'noradrenergic and selective serotonergic action' (NaSSA); and the atypical antidepressants including trazodone and mianserin.

Mechanism of action. Tricylics block reuptake of both noradrenaline and serotonin into the presynaptic neuron; SSRIs have a similar action on serotonin alone. MAOIs inhibit the breakdown of serotonin (and to a lesser extent noradrenaline) at the synapse. Mianserin and mirtazapine block presynaptic alpha 2 receptors. Any common mechanism of action for antidepressants probably involves modulation of pre- and/or post-synaptic receptors or electrophysiological responses.

Mode of administration. This is by mouth. Most antidepressants can be given once daily and are extensively and variably metabolized by first pass in the liver. The antidepressant response seldom occurs in less than 2 weeks and may not be fully apparent for 6 weeks. Patients not warned of the delayed therapeutic action are likely to be poorly compliant.

Indications. The main indication for antidepressants is depressive illness. Patients with biological features of depression but no delusions are likeliest to respond, but moderate to severe 'neurotic' depressions may also benefit. Most studies suggest a response rate of 60–70% (compared to 30% with placebo). Antidepressants are also useful in phobic anxiety, obsessive–compulsive neurosis and in preventing depressive relapse.

Side-effects. Include anticholinergic and antiadrenergic effects similar to those of the antipsychotics. In overdose they may trigger potentially fatal cardiac arrhythmias and seizures. Lofepramine is relatively safe in overdose and free of anticholinergic effects. SSRIs are largely devoid of tricyclic-like side-effects but may cause headache, anorexia and nausea. MAOIs (not moclobemide) can cause an occasionally fatal syndrome of hypertension and throbbing headache if foods containing large quantities of tyramine (e.g. cheese, red wine) are eaten.

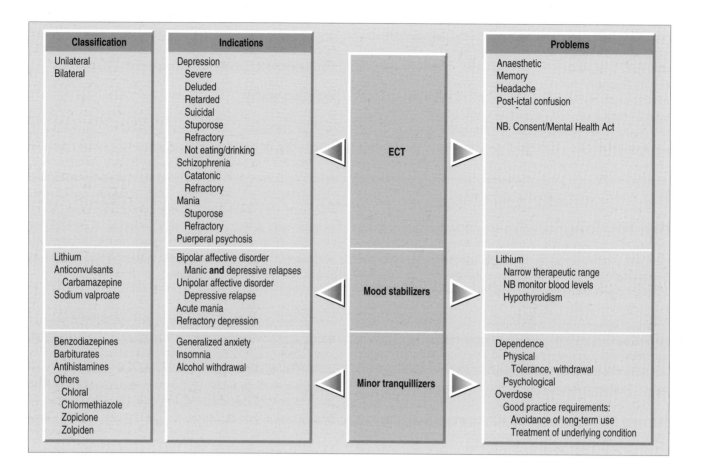

Classification	Indications		Problems

Unilateral
Bilateral
	Depression
	  Severe
	  Deluded
	  Retarded
	  Suicidal
	  Stuporose
	  Refractory
	  Not eating/drinking
	Schizophrenia
	  Catatonic
	  Refractory
	Mania
	  Stuporose
	  Refractory
	Puerperal psychosis
		ECT	Anaesthetic
			Memory
			Headache
			Post-ictal confusion
			
			NB. Consent/Mental Health Act

Lithium
Anticonvulsants
  Carbamazepine
Sodium valproate
	Bipolar affective disorder
	  Manic **and** depressive relapses
	Unipolar affective disorder
	  Depressive relapse
	Acute mania
	Refractory depression
		Mood stabilizers	Lithium
			  Narrow therapeutic range
			  NB monitor blood levels
			  Hypothyroidism

Benzodiazepines
Barbiturates
Antihistamines
Others
  Chloral
  Chlormethiazole
  Zopiclone
  Zolpiden
	Generalized anxiety
	Insomnia
	Alcohol withdrawal
		Minor tranquillizers	Dependence
			  Physical
			    Tolerance, withdrawal
			  Psychological
			Overdose
			  Good practice requirements:
			    Avoidance of long-term use
			    Treatment of underlying condition

ECT

Mechanism of action

ECT involves the induction of a modified epileptic seizure. A series of such treatments induces complex effects including neurotransmitter release; a transient increase in blood–brain barrier permeability; secretion of hypothalamic and pituitary hormones, and modulation of neurotransmitter receptors similar to those induced by antidepressant drugs.

Mode of administration

ECT is given two or three times a week, usually to a total of between four and 12 treatments. Before each treatment the patient is fasted for at least 4 hours, and is then given a short-acting anaesthetic, a muscle relaxant drug and a few seconds preoxygenation prior to the application of an electric current sufficient to trigger an epileptic seizure. This is given through electrodes placed bitemporally or with both on the non-dominant hemisphere. ECT can only be given if *either* the patient has given informed consent *or* is detained under the Mental Health Act and an independent consultant appointed by the Mental Health Act Commissioners agrees that ECT must

be given. In the latter situation, ECT can be initiated prior to the independent consultant's assessment under the provisions of Section 62 of the Mental Health Act.

Indications

The main indication for ECT is severe depression. Patients with depressive delusions and/or psychomotor retardation are likeliest to respond. Response rates may be as high as 90%. ECT should also be considered in depressed patients at high risk of suicide or not eating and drinking; those in whom other treatments have failed; in catatonic schizophrenia, in puerperal psychoses and in otherwise unresponsive schizophrenia or mania.

Contraindications

There are no absolute contraindications to ECT. Raised intracranial pressure, recent stroke, recent myocardial infarction and crescendo angina are important relative contraindications.

Side-effects

Side-effects include anaesthetic complications, dysrhythmias due to vagal stimulation, post-ictal headache and confusion, and retro- and anterograde amnesia with difficulties in registration and recall that may persist for several weeks. Memory problems are reduced by unilateral electrode placement which may, however, be slightly less effective.

Mood stabilizers

The most important of these is lithium (discussed below), although carbamazepine (which may be particularly useful in rapid-cycling bipolar illness) and sodium valproate are also used and there is some evidence for the efficacy of calcium channel blockers such as nifedipine.

Indications

The main indications for lithium are prophylaxis in recurrent affective disorder (unipolar and bipolar), acute treatment of mania and augmentation of antidepressants in resistant depression. Lithium may also be used in schizoaffective illness and in the control of aggression.

Mode of administration

Lithium is taken by mouth and excreted by the kidneys. It has a narrow therapeutic range (0.5–1.5 mmol/l). Prior to lithium therapy, thyroid and renal function should be evaluated. Serum lithium levels should be monitored regularly (initially weekly, thereafter every 12 weeks), blood being taken 8–12 hours after last dose. In patients on lithium, renal and thyroid function tests and in those on carbamazepine FBC should be monitored every 6 months. Patients should be warned that an unexplained sore throat may herald agranulocytosis.

Mechanism of action

Lithium interacts with all biological systems where sodium, potassium, calcium or magnesium are involved. At therapeutic blood levels it probably has effects on neurotransmission including 5HT, noradrenaline, dopamine and acetylchorine. Its interference with cAMP-linked receptors explains its action on the thyroid and kidney.

Side-effects and toxic effects

Side-effects of lithium include nausea, fine tremor, weight gain, oedema, polydipsia, polyuria, exacerbation of psoriasis and acne, and hypothyroidism. Toxicity is indicated by vomiting, diarrhoea, coarse tremor, slurred speech, ataxia, drowsiness, confusion, convulsions and coma. Treatment of toxicity/overdose involves cessation of lithium, forced diuresis (intravenous mannitol), haemodialysis or peritoneal dialysis. Carbamazepine may cause blood dyscrasias and rashes.

Contraindications

Lithium should be avoided in renal, cardiac, thyroid and Addison's disease and in pregnancy and breastfeeding. Dehydration and diuretics can lead to lithium toxicity. Adverse interactions can also occur between lithium and non-steroidal anti-inflammatory drugs, calcium channel blockers and some antibiotics. Carbamazepine is also teratogenic and may interfere with the action of oral contraceptives, necessitating other contraceptive precautions.

Minor tranquillizers

The most important of these are the benzodiazepines (BDZs), although these were preceded by the barbiturates and chloral hydrate.

Drugs currently in use and indications

As the BDZs are anxiolytic, sleep inducing, anticonvulsant and muscle relaxants, their indications include insomnia, generalised (but not phobic) anxiety, alcohol withdrawal states and the control of violent behaviour. Underlying conditions (such as depression) should always be excluded and behavioural alternative treatments considered. BDZs are also used as 'second-line' drugs in refractory epilepsy. Chlormethiazole, zopiclone, zolpiden and antihistamines such as promethazine may be used as hypnotics. Buspirone has anxiolytic effects.

Mode of administration

The main mode of administration is oral, but IM, IV or rectal administration may be required in status epilepticus and in violent patients.

Pharmacokinetics

Most have active metabolites, some with half-lives of several days. The long-acting BDZs include diazepam, chlordiazepoxide and nitrazepam; lorazepam, oxazepam and temazepam are shorter acting BDZs.

Mechanism of action

Mechanism of action of BDZs and most other minor tranquillizers (apart from antihistamines) is potentiation of the inhibitory effects of GABA.

Toxic and side-effects

Toxic effects and side-effects of minor tranquillizers include drowsiness, sedation, ataxia, respiratory depression and disinhibition which may lead (paradoxically) to aggression. Tolerance to BDZs frequently occurs, and there is a prolonged withdrawal syndrome, with marked anxiety, shakiness, abdominal cramps, perceptual disturbances, persecutory delusions and fits. They should therefore usually only be prescribed for no more than a couple of weeks. Weaning patients off BZDs to which they have (iatrogenically) become dependent may take months or even years.

Contraindications

BDZs potentiate alcohol and other minor tranquillizers; the combination is dangerous in overdose.

35 Cross-cultural psychiatry

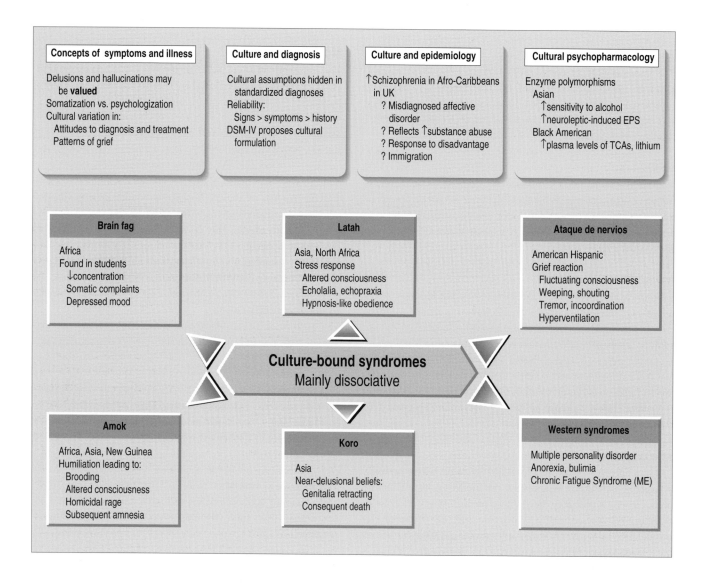

Concepts of symptoms and illness

Delusions and hallucinations may be **valued**
Somatization vs. psychologization
Cultural variation in:
   Attitudes to diagnosis and treatment
   Patterns of grief

Culture and diagnosis

Cultural assumptions hidden in standardized diagnoses
Reliability:
   Signs > symptoms > history
DSM-IV proposes cultural formulation

Culture and epidemiology

↑Schizophrenia in Afro-Caribbeans in UK
   ? Misdiagnosed affective disorder
   ? Reflects ↑substance abuse
   ? Response to disadvantage
   ? Immigration

Cultural psychopharmacology

Enzyme polymorphisms
   Asian
      ↑sensitivity to alcohol
      ↑neuroleptic-induced EPS
   Black American
      ↑plasma levels of TCAs, lithium

Brain fag

Africa
Found in students
   ↓concentration
   Somatic complaints
   Depressed mood

Latah

Asia, North Africa
Stress response
   Altered consciousness
   Echolalia, echopraxia
   Hypnosis-like obedience

Ataque de nervios

American Hispanic
Grief reaction
   Fluctuating consciousness
   Weeping, shouting
   Tremor, incoordination
   Hyperventilation

Culture-bound syndromes
Mainly dissociative

Amok

Africa, Asia, New Guinea
Humiliation leading to:
   Brooding
   Altered consciousness
   Homicidal rage
   Subsequent amnesia

Koro

Asia
Near-delusional beliefs:
   Genitalia retracting
   Consequent death

Western syndromes

Multiple personality disorder
Anorexia, bulimia
Chronic Fatigue Syndrome (ME)

Culture is the way that different groups of people conceptualize and perceive their world and interact with their environment. It incorporates patterns of social and family relationships and religious beliefs. Cross-cultural psychiatry examines concepts of mental health and illness, their underlying causes and how symptomatology is culturally determined. It addresses issues of the universality and prevalence of psychiatric diagnoses, their treatments and their prognoses.

Concepts of symptoms, illness and healing

Our judgements concerning 'abnormal' mental symptoms or disease states frequently contain cultural assumptions of which we are unaware. The examples below are intended to make readers more critical of their own judgements.

Hallucinations and delusions of control are two of the clearest manifestations of mental illness within western culture. In contrast, among the Xhosa of Southern Africa, hallucinations carry status. More generally, 'possession states' (brief experiences of external control deliberately induced by ritual and/or drugs), are regarded as normal and indeed valued in most cultures.

A further example of the 'oddity' of our western perspective is insistence on the 'mind/body' dualism. Rather than dismiss the bodily symptoms (common to many 'culture-bound' syndromes) within what we consider 'mental illness' as 'somatization', we might more appropriately regard purely 'mental' symptoms (e.g. depression, anxiety) as manifestations of Western 'psychologization'.

Cultural attitudes to death and loss are particularly important in interpreting an individual's experience of bereavement (see Chapter 8). Stages of 'normal' grieving may be very different in, for example, Great Britain, India and Greece and cultural norms cannot be ignored in diagnosing 'abnormal' grief reactions.

The attribution of abnormal personality (see Chapter 12) is particularly dependent on cultural norms. For example, within western countries, the 'antisocial' personality may be understandable and even have survival value in individuals from deprived inner-city areas with chronic exposure to violent crime, particularly where these are not offset by a stable family environment.

Culture may also influence attitudes to healing, a concept which is wider in non-western societies, taking into account kinship relationships and links with the supernatural world. Elaborate rituals are often involved; the 'ward round' may be seen as a Western equivalent. Acceptance of treatment implies a shared belief in illness and in the legitimacy of intervention. For example, some Christian sects may accept conventional diagnoses but nonetheless oppose treatment as an 'artificial' intervention with God's will.

Culture and standardized diagnosis

The Kraepelinian approach to psychiatric diagnosis and classification (see Chapter 2), itself a reflection of western culture rather than culture-independent, remains central to ICD-10 and DSM-IV. It relies on the elicitation of patterns of symptoms and signs that are brought together to make 'reliable' diagnoses. The 'reliability' (or reproducibility) of such symptoms and signs is, however, questionable. The World Health Organization carried out a cross-cultural investigation of the process of psychiatric diagnosis, the International Pilot Study on Schizophrenia (IPSS), in the 1960s and 1970s. The IPSS showed that, although psychotic symptoms (delusions and hallucinations) elicited from individual patient interviews showed satisfactory reliability, clinical signs (e.g. incongruous or flat affect) were much less reliable, and corroborative evidence (family, work and social background) less so still. At diagnostic level, psychotic disorders (including psychotic depression as well as schizophrenia) could be identified reliably, but neurotic and dissociative diagnoses were much less secure. It is noteworthy that many so-called 'culture-bound' syndromes have dissociative features.

As a step towards the recognition of these issues, DSM-IV (although retaining multiple cultural assumptions within the axes of 'psychosocial and environmental problems' and 'global functioning') contains an 'outline' for 'cultural formulation'.

Culture and epidemiology

The IPSS established that the prevalence of schizophrenia was remarkably stable across cultures, although its prognosis was better in non-Western societies. This may reflect greater availability of home support without high expressed emotion and the absence of a stigmatising 'label' of chronic schizophrenia. In contrast, the prevalence of depression was much more variable and its presentation in non-Western groups was often with somatic symptoms. Even for schizophrenia, cultural factors within a multicultural society may influence prevalence. For example, in the UK, an excess prevalence of schizophrenia is reported among Afro-Caribbeans. This may reflect several factors including misdiagnosis of affective disorders as schizophrenia, errors in estimating the total Afro-Caribbean population, cultural patterns of substance misuse (including a high prevalence of cannabis-(Ganja) induced psychoses), the complex interaction between immigration and mental illness (although the excess is also apparent in 'second generation' Afro-Caribbeans) and mental illness being an intelligible response to disadvantage.

Pharmacological response across cultures

Racial differences in distribution of enzyme polymorphisms are reflected in, for example, increased sensitivity to alcohol (and decreased prevalence of alcohol dependence) in people of Asian origin, who also appear more susceptible to drug-induced dyskinesias. Similarly, black Americans tend to develop higher plasma levels for given doses of tricyclic antidepressants and lithium than their white counterparts, with resultantly increased sensitivity to both therapeutic and adverse affects.

Culture-bound syndromes

According to DSM-IV, these denote locality-specific patterns of abnormal behaviour or troubling experience. Many have been described, mostly representing somatic and/or dissociative responses to stress. A few of the better known are outlined below.

Amok, described in Africa, Asia and New Guinea, is a response to humiliation involving initial brooding followed by a period of altered consciousness with uncontrollable (usually homicidal and sometimes suicidal) rage, for which the subject has no subsequent memory. Traditionally, surviving sufferers were immune from legal redress, much as the French *crime passionnel*.

Ataque de nervios occurs in American Hispanic groups, and consists of a grief reaction characterized by fluctuating conscious level (often with subsequent amnesia), crying, shouting, trembling and difficulty in moving limbs. Hyperventilation may be important in precipitating symptoms.

Latah, which occurs in Asia and North Africa, is a response to intense stress characterized by altered consciousness, hyper-suggestibility and mimicry (including echolalia and echopraxia).

Koro, found mainly in Asia, involves intense anxiety centred on the belief that one's genitalia are retracting and that their disappearance will result in death. The traditional management is to tie a string around the penis and pull. Koro is associated with local tradition that ghosts have no genitals and is thus not delusional.

Brain fag is found mainly in African students, and is characterized by concentration difficulties, vague somatic complaints and depressed mood.

Some 'Western' syndromes, including multiple personality disorder, anorexia nervosa, bulimia nervosa and chronic fatigue syndrome (ME) may also be considered 'culture-bound'.

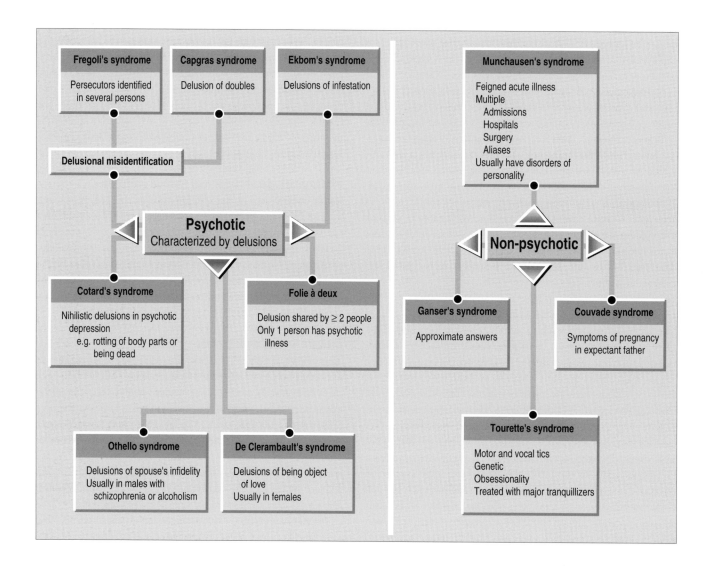

The features of the best described syndromes are summarized below, although it must be borne in mind that most have not been studied systematically. They can conveniently be divided into psychotic (characterized by delusions and hallucinations) and non-psychotic syndromes.

Psychotic

Delusional misidentification syndrome (DMS)

Several types of this syndrome have been described; the best known are the syndromes of *Capgras* and *Fregoli*. The Capgras' syndrome was first described in 1923 by Capgras and Reboul-Lachaux and is now recognized as a psychotic state characterized by a delusion in which the patient believes that a person has been replaced by an exact double. In contrast, the rarer Fregoli's syndrome involves the delusion that the patient's persecutors are

masquerading as his/her attendants (such as the doctor or nurse). DMS can occur in schizophrenia, affective disorders and acute organic confusional states. Treatment is of the primary disorder.

Delusional parasitosis

Delusional parasitosis (DP) is also known as Ekbom's syndrome (although the term is also used to describe a neurological syndrome of 'restless legs'). Sufferers (F/M ratio 3 : 1) believe that insects are colonizing their body, particularly the skin and eyes. Initial presentation is often to public health workers (with persistent demands for deinfestation) or to dermatologists or infectious disease physicians, with importuning and bizarre requests for investigation and treatment. Delusions may be circumscribed or part of a schizophrenic or depressive illness. Antipsychotics and/or antidepressants are the mainstay of treatment.

Folie à deux

Folie à deux consists of a delusional belief that is shared by two or more people (usually within a family), of whom only one has other psychotic features. The pair are often isolated from others in terms of distance or due to cultural or language barriers. The delusion is usually persecutory or hypochondriacal, and the psychotic individual (principal) tends to be more intelligent and better educated, and has a dominating influence over the non-psychotic (more submissive) recipient(s). Diagnosis of the principal is most commonly schizophrenia but may be an affective disorder or dementia, and primary treatment is of the underlying condition. A period of separation, followed by supportive individual and/or family therapy focussed on the recipient may be helpful.

De Clerambault's syndrome (erotomania)

The patient (usually female) has the unfounded and delusional belief that someone (usually a man of higher social status) is in love with her. The patient makes inappropriate advances to the object of her passion and becomes angry (and sometimes violent) when rejected. The syndrome may exist in isolation, or as part of an affective (usually manic) disorder or, more rarely, schizophrenia. When men are affected they present a greater forensic problem. Management frequently involves hospitalization (sometimes compulsory) to prevent harassment or injury. Underlying conditions should be treated as appropriate; where none is identified neuroleptics may be useful.

Othello syndrome

Othello syndrome (OS, morbid jealousy) may complicate long-term alcohol abuse, and is also sometimes found in severe depression. The patient, usually male, is delusionally convinced that his spouse is being unfaithful. He goes to great lengths to produce 'evidence' of the infidelity (e.g. stains on under-clothes/sheets) and to extract a confession. Paradoxically, the spouse is sometimes driven to true infidelity. There is a substantial risk of violence (even homicide); thus, distant separation may be warranted and compulsory hospitalization and treatment is often necessary. It tends to occur with a new partner.

Cotard's syndrome

Cotard's syndrome is characterized by 'nihilistic' delusions, in which the patient believes that parts of his/her body are decaying or rotting, or have ceased to exist. Patients may also believe themselves to be already dead, or (paradoxically) unable to die. Although the syndrome is almost invariably found in the context of psychotic depression, the nihilistic ideas themselves often have a grandiose flavour (e.g. the world will end because of them). ECT is usually the treatment of first choice.

Non-psychotic
Tourette's syndrome (TS)

TS was originally described by Jean Itard in 1825 but named after George Gilles de la Tourette, a French neuropsychiatrist who described nine cases in 1885, emphasizing the triad of multiple tics, echolalia and coprolalia. Current research suggests that TS is not really rare; the cited prevalence of 1/2000 is an underestimate. Males are more often affected (3–4 : 1). The family history is frequently positive. TS usually begins with facial tics such as excessive blinking; the median age at onset is 7 years. Associated features include ADHD and OCB. Treatment is with antipsychotics (for tics and OCB/OCD), clonidine (for ADHD) and SSRIs.

Munchausen's syndrome

Munchausen's syndrome is also known as Factitious disorder and is characterized by deliberately feigned symptomatology, usually physical (e.g. abdominal pain), but can be psychiatric (e.g. hallucinations, multiple bereavements or sexual abuse). Occasionally, the disorder can be by proxy, as when a mother fakes illnesses in her child (MSBP). These result in multiple presentations to casualty departments, usually to several hospitals, with frequent admissions often culminating in surgical procedures. Patients often use multiple aliases, are often of no fixed abode and usually have no regular GP. When discovered, the patients usually discharge themselves against medical advice. The syndrome characteristically occurs in the setting of a severely disordered personality. Management is difficult, although confrontation without rejection may prove helpful.

Couvade syndrome

Couvade syndrome consists of the experience of symptoms resembling those of pregnancy (abdominal swelling and/or spasms, nausea and vomiting, etc.) in expectant fathers. Anxiety and psychosomatic symptoms (e.g. toothache) are common. The prevalence of mild forms is as high as 20%. The condition (which in some cultures is quite acceptable and may even be expected) is usually self-limiting and responds to counselling but often recurs in subsequent pregnancies.

Ganser's syndrome (GS)

The central feature of this syndrome is the giving of approximate, absurd and often inconsistent answers to simple questions. The patient may say $2 + 2 = 5$, or, when asked the colour of snow, reply 'green'. The syndrome is also characterized by clouding of consciousness, true and/or pseudo-hallucinations (visual or auditory) and features of somatic conversion (see Chapter 25). In pure form, GS represents a dissociative reaction of defence against intolerable stress, although there may be an underlying depression warranting treatment in its own right. GS is overrepresented in prison populations. Spontaneous improvement often occurs, and is characteristically accompanied by amnesia for the abnormal behaviour. Recovery may be hastened by admission to hospital and psychotherapeutic exploration of underlying conflicts.

Further reading

Chapters 1 and 2

Sims, A. (1995) *Symptoms in the Mind*. 2nd ed. W.B. Saunders.

WHO (1992) *The ICD-10 Classification of Mental and Behavioural Disorders*. World Health Organisation, Geneva.

APA (1994) *Diagnostic and Statistical Manual of Mental Disorder*. 4th ed. American Psychiatric Association, Washington DC.

Chapters 3 and 4

DeQuardo, J.R. (1998) Pharmacologic treatment of first-episode schizophrenia: Early intervention is key to outcome. *Journal of Clinical Psychiatry* **59**, SUPPL. 19, 9–17.

Riecher-Rossler, A. & Rossler, W. (1998) The course of schizophrenic psychoses: what do we really know? A selective review from an epidemiological perspective. *European Archives of Psychiatry and Clinical Neuroscience* **248**, 189–202.

DeLisi, L.E. (1999) A critical overview of recent investigations into the genetics of schizophrenia. *Current Opinion in Psychiatry* **12**, 29–39.

Chapter 5

Akiskal, H.S. (1997) Overview of chronic depressions and their clinical management. In: *Dysthymia and the Spectrum of Chronic Depressions* (Akiskal, H.S. & Cassano, G.B. (eds)) pp 1–34. The Guilford Press, New York.

Ronalds, C., Creed, F., Stone, K. *et al.* (1997) Outcome of anxiety and depressive disorders in primary care. *British Journal of Psychiatry* **171**, 427–433.

Zisook, S., Paulus, M., Shuchter, S.R. & Judd, L.L. (1997) The many faces of depression following spousal bereavement. *Journal of Affective Disorders* **45**, 85–94.

Wolpert, L. (1998) *Malignant Sadness*. Faber.

Chapter 6

Schou, M. (1998) The effect of prophylactic lithium treatment on mortality and suicidal behavior: a review for clinicians. *Journal of Affective Disorder* **50**, 253–259.

Tannock, C. Mania and bipolar disorder: Current concepts on assessment, diagnosis and management. *International Journal of Psychiatry in Clinical Practice* **2**, 97–105.

Chapter 7

Hawton, K., Fagg, J., Simkin, S., Bale, E. & Bond, A. (1997) Trends in deliberate self-harm in Oxford, 1985–1995. Implications for clinical services and the prevention of suicide. *British Journal of Psychiatry* **171**, 556–560.

Harris, E.C. & Barraclough, B. (1997) Excess mortality of mental disorder. *British Journal of Psychiatry* **173**, 11–53.

Hawton, K., Arensman, E., Townsend, E. *et al.* (1998). Deliberate self harm: Systematic review of efficacy of psychosocial and pharmacological treatments in preventing repetition. *British Medical Journal* **317**, 441–447.

Chapter 8

Yehuda, R. (1998) Psychoneuroendocrinology of post-traumatic stress disorder. *Psychiatric Clinics of North America* **21**, 359–379.

Turnbull, G.J. (1998) A review of post–traumatic stress disorder. Part I: Historical development and classification. *Injury*. **29**, 87–91.

Turnbull, G.J. (1998) A review of post–traumatic stress disorder. Part II: Treatment. *Injury*. 260, **29**, 169–175.

Chapter 9

Simon, N. & Pollack, M. (1998) Current status and future prospects for anxiolytic drug therapy. *Primary Care Psychiatry* **4**, 157–167.

Hoehn-Saric, R. (1998) Generalised anxiety disorder. Guidelines for diagnosis and treatment. *CNS-Drugs*. **9**, 85–98.

Chapter 10

Miguel, E.C., Rauch, S.L. & Jenike, M.A. (1997) Obsessive-compulsive disorder. *Psychiatric Clinics of North America* **20**, 863–883.

Skoog, G. & Skoog, I. (1999) A 40-year follow-up of patients with obsessive-compulsive disorder. *Archives of General Psychiatry* **56**, 121–127.

Chapter 11

Steiner, H. & Lock, J. (1998) Anorexia nervosa and bulimia nervosa in children and adolescents: A review of the past 10 years. *Journal of the American Academy of Child and Adolescent Psychiatry* **37**, 352–359.

Troop, N.A., Holbrey, A. & Treasure, J.L. (1998) Stress, coping, and crisis support in eating disorders. *International Journal of Eating Disorders* **24**, 157–166.

Chapter 12

Dolan, B. & Coid, J. (1994) *Psychopathic & Antisocial Personality Disorders: Treatment & Research Issues*. Gaskell Press, London.

Tyrer, P. (1994) What are the borders of borderline personality disorder? *Acta Psychiatrica Scandanavia* SUPPL. **379**, 38–44.

Tyrer, P., Gunderson, J., Lyons, M. & Tohen, M. (1997) Extent of comorbidity between mental state and personality disorders. *Journal of Personality Disorders* **11**, 242–259.

Chapters 13 and 14

Ghodse, H. (1995) *Drug and Addiction Behaviour. A Guide to Treatment*. 2nd ed. Blackwell Science, Oxford.

Department of Health. (1999) *Drug Misuse and Dependence—Guidelines on Clinical Management*. HMSO.

Rassool, G.H. (1998) *Substance Use and Misuse: Nature, Context and Clinical Interventions*. Blackwell Science, Oxford.

Chapter 15

Barry, S. (1997) Depression in pregnancy and childbirth. In: *Depression and Physical Illness* (Robertson, M.M. and Katona, C.L.E. (eds)) pp 115–132. John Wiley and Sons, Chichester.

Pound, A. & Abel, K. (1996) Motherhood and mental illness. In: *Planning Community Mental Health Services for Women* (Abel, K. *et al.* (eds)) pp 20–36. Routledge.

Chapter 16

Watkin, V. & Katona, C. (1998) Functional psychiatric illness in old age. In: *Geriatric Medicine and Gerontology*, 5th edition (Tallis, R., Fillit, H., Brocklehurst, J.C. (eds)) pp 741–755. Churchill Livingstone, Edinburgh.

Chapter 17

Macdonald, A.J.D. (1998) Delirium. In: *Geriatric Medicine and Gerontology*, 5th edition (Tallis, R., Fillit, H., Brocklehurst, J.C. (eds)) pp 685–699. Churchill Livingstone, Edinburgh.

Chapter 18

Russell, E.M. & Burns, A. (1998) Dementia: Clinical presentation and management. In: *Geriatric Medicine and Gerontology*, 5th edition (Tallis, R., Fillit, H., Brocklehurst, J.C. (eds)) pp 727–740. Churchill Livingstone, Edinburgh.

Chapters 19 and 20

Sanders, R.D. & Keshavan, M.S. (1998) The neurologic examination in adult psychiatry: From soft signs to hard science. *Journal of Neuropsychiatry and Clinical Neurosciences* **230**, 395–404.

Frumin, M., Chisholm, T., Dickey, C.C. & Daffner, K.R. (1998) Psychiatric and behavioral problems. *Neurologic Clinics* **16**, 521–544.

Obeso, J.A. *et al.* (1997) Basal ganglia pathophysiology: a critical review. *Advances in Neurology* **74**, 3–18.

Chapters 20 and 22

Cassidy, L.J. & Jellinek, M.S. (1998) Approaches to recognition and management of childhood psychiatric disorders in pediatric primary care. *Pediatric Clinics of North America* **45**, 1037–1052.

Chapter 23

Berenson, C.K. (1998) Frequently missed diagnoses in adolescent psychiatry. *Psychiatric Clinics of North America* **21**, 917–926.

Chapter 24

Russell, O. (Ed) (1997) *Seminars in the Psychiatry of Learning Disabilities*. Royal College of Psychiatrists and Gaskell Press, London.

Chapter 25

Gjaerum, B. & Blomhoff, S. (1998) Assessment of the mental state in medically ill adults. *Current Opinion in Psychiatry* **11**, 643–647.

Antonowicz, J.L. (1998) Missed diagnoses in consultation liaison psychiatry. *Psychiatric Clinics of North America* **21/3**, 705–714.

Chapter 26

Thornicroft, G., Wykes, T., Holloway, F., Johnson, S. & Szmukler, G. (1998) From efficacy to effectiveness in community mental health services. PRiSM psychosis study 10. *British Journal of Psychiatry* **173**, 423–427.

Burns, T. & Bristow, M. (1997) The role of the GP in the management of schizophrenia. *Primary-Care-Psychiatry* **3**, 169–173.

Chapter 27

Exworthy, T. (1998) Institutions and services in forensic psychiatry. *Journal of Forensic Psychiatry* **9**, 395–412.

Taylor, P.J., Gunn, J. (1999) Homicides by people with mental illness: Myth and reality *British Journal of Psychiatry* **174**, 9–14.

Chapter 28

Jones, R. (Ed) (1994) *Mental Health Act Manual*. Sweet & Maxwell.

Chapter 29

Royal College of Psychiatrists (1998). *The Management of Imminent Violence*. Gaskell Press.

Chapter 30

Leiblum, S.R. (1998) Definition and classification of female sexual disorders. *International Journal of Impotence Research* **10**, SUPPL. 2, S104–S106.

Chapter 31

Pajonk, F.G. & Naber, D. (1998) Human immunodeficiency virus and mental disorders *Current Opinion in Psychiatry* **11**, 305–310.

Chapter 32

Salkovskis, P.M., Forrester, E. & Richards, C. (1998) Cognitive-behavioural approach to understanding obsessional thinking. *British Journal of Psychiatry* **173**, SUPPL. 35, 53–63.

Rycroft, C. (1995) *A Critical Dictionary of Psychoanalysis*. Penguin.

Chapters 33 and 34

Cookson, J., Taylor, D. & Katona, C. (in press) *Drugs in Psychiatry*. Gaskell Press.

Nemeroff, C.B. (1998) Psychopharmacology of affective disorders in the 21st Century. *Biological Psychiatry* **44**, 515–517.

Cooper, S.J., Ingram, R. (1998) Electroconvulsive therapy in current psychiatric practice. *Primary Care Psychiatry* **4**, 169–178.

Fleischhacker, W. (1999) The psychopharmacology of schizophrenia. *Current Opinion in Psychiatry* **103:12**, 53–59.

Chapter 35

Littlewood, R. & Lipsedge, M. (1997) *Aliens & Alienists: Ethnic Minorities & Psychiatry*. 3rd ed. Routledge.

Chapter 36

Asher, R. (1951) Munchausen's syndrome. *Lancet I*, 339–341.

Enoch, M.D. (1991) *Uncommon Psychiatric Syndromes*. Butterworth.

Robertson, M.M. (1994) Annotation: Gills de la Tourette syndrome—an update. *Journal of Child Psychology and Psychiatry* **35**, 597–611.

Questions

The following multiple choice questions are intended to help readers check their understanding of the material covered in the book and to aid revision. They are arranged by subject matter and their sequence corresponds with that of the chapters to which they refer.

1 Important factors to be considered in assessing a patient's speech include:
(a) Rate
(b) Pressure
(c) Tone
(d) Coherence
(e) Perspicacity

2 Abnormal beliefs include:
(a) Obsessions
(b) Phobias
(c) Ideas of reference
(d) Autochthonous delusions
(e) Depersonalization

3 Main ways of classifying mental disorders include:
(a) Categorical
(b) Dimensional
(c) Multiaxial
(d) Symptomatic
(e) Pragmatic

4 ICD-10:
(a) Uses operational definitions
(b) Is reliant on clinical description
(c) Measures personality disorders on Axis II
(d) Excludes organic disorders
(e) Is published by the World Health Organisation

5 Schnieider's first rank symptoms of schizophrenia include:
(a) Thought echo
(b) Thought block
(c) Delusional perception
(d) Olfactory hallucinations
(e) Somatic passivity

6 Abnormal family processes implicated in schizophrenia include:
(a) Oversubmissive mother
(b) Low expressed emotion
(c) Ambivalence
(d) Early parental separation
(e) Adverse life events

7 Factors predictive of a good prognosis in schizophrenia include:
(a) Insidious onset
(b) A strong affective component
(c) Older age at onset
(d) Predominantly 'positive' symptoms
(e) Positive family history

8 Psychosocial factors implicated in the aetiology of depression include:
(a) Unemployment
(b) Being an only child
(c) Overstimulation
(d) Childhood abuse
(e) High serotonin levels

9 Recognised depressive subtypes include:
(a) Catatonic
(b) Dysthymic
(c) Bipolar
(d) Atypical
(e) Borderline

10 Mania:
(a) Has a recurrence rate of about 20% in 10 years
(b) Is characterized by irritability
(c) Is associated with first rank symptoms in 25% of cases
(d) Is characterized by nihilistic delusions
(e) May be treated with carbamazepine

11 The following statements about the epidemiology of mania are true:
(a) The typical age of onset is in the mid teens
(b) Lifetime risk is about 5%
(c) It is commoner in women
(d) It is commoner in higher socioeconomic groups
(e) Incidence is about 20 per 100,000 per year

12 Factors associated with a markedly increased risk of suicide include:
(a) Drug abuse
(b) Generalized anxiety
(c) Unemployment
(d) Availability of firearms
(e) House move

13 Factors associated with a markedly increased risk of deliberate self harm include:
(a) Male gender
(b) Lower socioeconomic class
(c) Living with a partner
(d) Personality disorder
(e) Age >50

14 Features indicative of atypical grief include:
(a) Early onset
(b) Rapid progression
(c) Despair
(d) Guilt
(e) Shock

15 Post-traumatic stress disorder:
  (a) Is usually associated with anxiety symptoms
  (b) More frequently occurs following natural than 'man-made' disasters
  (c) Is always self-limiting
  (d) Responds well to benzodiazepines
  (e) Can be treated with cognitive-behavioural therapy (CBT)

16 Characteristic clinical features of generalized anxiety disorder include:
  (a) Apprehensive expectations
  (b) Hypovigilance
  (c) Fear of going crazy
  (d) Muscle tension
  (e) Autonomic arousal

17 Recognised treatments of anxiety disorders include:
  (a) Cognitive behavioural therapy (CBT)
  (b) Monoamine oxidase inhibitors
  (c) Maintenance benzodiazepines
  (d) Carbamazepine
  (e) Interpersonal Psychotherapy (IPT)

18 The following is true about obsessive-compulsive disorder (OCD):
  (a) It occurs more frequently in women
  (b) It is characterized by delusions of contamination
  (c) It is associated with dopaminergic underactivity
  (d) It responds well to psychoanalysis
  (e) The lifetime risk is 10%

19 Bulimia nervosa:
  (a) Is characterized by carbohydrate starvation
  (b) Occurs with a female : male ratio of 3 : 1
  (c) Carries a better prognosis if the patient is underweight
  (d) May be associated with transient trance-like states
  (e) Is characterised by the presence of lanugo hair

20 Anorexia nervosa:
  (a) Carries a 10% risk of suicide
  (b) Is associated with tachycardia
  (c) Often presents in the early teenage years
  (d) Is seldom associated with binge eating
  (e) May cause life-threatening hypokalaemia

21 The following statements about borderline personality disorder are true:
  (a) It may be known as anankastic personality disorder
  (b) Binge eating sometimes occurs
  (c) Hallucinations may be present
  (d) Sufferers usually show little interest in sex
  (e) Response to antidepressants is sometimes good

22 Established treatments of personality disorders include:
  (a) Dynamic psychotherapy
  (b) Therapeutic community
  (c) Limit setting
  (d) Methylphenidate
  (e) Electroconvulsive therapy

23 Cardinal features of drug dependence include:
  (a) Intolerance
  (b) Reduced social activity
  (c) Neglect of other interests
  (d) Hallucinations
  (e) Somatic passivity

24 Physical features of opiate withdrawal include:
  (a) Mydriasis
  (b) Tremor
  (c) Diarrhoea
  (d) Piloerection
  (e) Bradycardia

25 Alcohol dependence:
  (a) Is frequently associated with a microcytic anaemia
  (b) Is frequently associated with an elevated gamma-glutamyl transferase level
  (c) Is associated with atrophy of Wernicke's area
  (d) May be treated by group psychotherapy
  (e) Carries an increased risk of complex partial seizures

26 Management of alcohol withdrawal includes:
  (a) Chlorpromazine to reduce risk of seizures
  (b) Ascorbic acid supplementation
  (c) Frequent changes of nursing staff
  (d) Disulfiram
  (e) Cognitive behavioural therapy

27 Postpartum psychosis:
  (a) Occurs after 1% of deliveries
  (b) Is usually affective
  (c) Mandates cessation of breastfeeding
  (d) Occurs more frequently following instrumental delivery
  (e) Seldom responds to ECT

28 Non-psychotic depression after childbirth:
  (a) Usually presents within the first postpartum week
  (b) Is seldom associated with suicidal intent
  (c) Is usually inherited
  (d) Is associated with a history of premenstrual tension
  (e) Can be treated with antidepressants

29 Depression in old age:
  (a) Carries a low risk of suicide
  (b) Often presents with somatic symptoms
  (c) May present as a dementia
  (d) Seldom responds to electroconvulsive therapy
  (e) Is more often associated with anxiety symptoms than depression earlier in life

30 The following statements concerning mania in old age are true:
  (a) It occurs more frequently in women
  (b) It may be associated with prominent subjective confusion
  (c) Elation occurs less frequently than in younger people
  (d) It may be precipitated by stroke
  (e) Response to lithium is poor

31 Characteristic clinical features of delirium include:
(a) Confusion worst at night
(b) Apathy
(c) Illusions
(d) Consistent cognitive deficits
(e) Hypervigilance

32 Features of delirium which help distinguish it from dementia include:
(a) Insidious onset
(b) Presence of delusions
(c) Tactile hallucinations
(d) Clouding of consciousness
(e) Flight of ideas

33 Conditions which may be mistaken for dementia include:
(a) Normal ageing
(b) Depression
(c) Myxoedema
(d) Othello syndrome
(e) Delirium

34 The following statements concerning Alzheimer's Disease are true:
(a) Periventricular lucencies are often found on CT scan
(b) Dopaminergic neurotransmission is markedly reduced
(c) Risk is increased in people homozygous for the E4 allele of the apolipoprotein gene
(d) Hypertension is common
(e) Sleep is often disrupted

35 Huntington's Disease:
(a) Is associated with decreased GABAergic neurotransmission
(b) Has autosomal recessive inheritance
(c) The determining gene is localized on Chromosome 4
(d) Carries a 25% risk of dementia
(e) Is associated with nucleus accumbens degeneration

36 Psychiatric complications of Parkinson's Disease include:
(a) Frontal impairment
(b) Iatrogenic psychosis
(c) Depression
(d) Korsakoff's syndrome
(e) Obsessions

37 The following statements are true about epilepsy:
(a) Treatment with phenobarbitone may cause depression
(b) Schizophreniform psychoses are associated with a left-sided temporal seizure focus
(c) Mania is common
(d) Risk of suicide is increased most markedly in absence seizures
(e) Pseudo-seizures may occur

38 Hypothyroidism may present as:
(a) Asperger's syndrome
(b) Dementia
(c) Depression
(d) Anxiety
(e) Anorexia

39 The following features of truancy help to distinguish it from school refusal:
(a) The whereabouts of the child during school hours are not known
(b) Anxiety symptoms are prominent
(c) Comorbid conduct disorder
(d) Good academic performance
(e) Cyclothymic personality

40 The following statements about child abuse are true:
(a) The presentation may be of Munchausen's Syndrome by proxy
(b) Victims are usually of low birthweight
(c) There is frequently a history of early maternal separation
(d) Abusing parents have themselves often been abused
(e) Social Class I is overrepresented

41 Attention-deficit hyperactivity disorder in childhood:
(a) Is commoner in boys
(b) Is characterized by grandiosity
(c) May be treated with dexamphetamine
(d) Seldom persists into adult life
(e) May be predictive of adult antisocial personality disorder

42 Clinical features of autism include:
(a) Impaired language development
(b) Hemiparesis
(c) Ritualistic behaviours
(d) Auditory hallucinations
(e) Aloofness

43 Conduct disorder in adolescence:
(a) Often coexists with substance abuse
(b) Is seldom associated with criminal behaviour
(c) Is more common in females
(d) May respond to family therapy
(e) Is often associated with depressive symptoms

44 The following statements are true about schizophrenia in adolescence:
(a) Onset is commonly before the age of 15
(b) The presentation may be with deteriorating school performance
(c) Social withdrawal is rare
(d) Schneiderian first-rank symptoms may be fleeting
(e) Extrapyramidal reactions to neuroleptics are rare

45 Characteristic features of Down's Syndrome include:
(a) High arched feet
(b) Cardiac septal defects
(c) Multiple palmar creases
(d) Hyperthyroidism
(e) Flat occiput

46 Common psychiatric complications of learning disability include:
(a) Conversion symptoms
(b) Hallucinations
(c) Phobic anxiety
(d) Depressed mood
(e) Primary delusional perception

47 Testamentary capacity requires:
(a) IQ >90
(b) Understanding the value of one's property
(c) Understanding what a will is
(d) The absence of mental illness
(e) Understanding who might have a legitimate claim on one's property

48 Significant associations between crime and mental illness include:
(a) Depression and shoplifting
(b) Puerperal psychosis and infanticide
(c) Borderline personality disorder and homicide
(d) Learning disability and arson
(e) Alcohol dependence and driving offences

49 The cluster of clinical features of schizophrenia described by Bleuler include:
(a) Affective incongruity
(b) Ambivalence
(c) Anhedonia
(d) Agitation
(e) Autochthonous delusions

50 Symptoms triggering referral of medical patients for psychiatric opinion include:
(a) Chronic pain
(b) Fatigue
(c) Agitation
(d) Confusion
(e) Aggressivity

51 Depression in a physically ill patient frequently presents with:
(a) Suicidal threats
(b) Guilt
(c) Fatigue
(d) Requests for antidepressants
(e) Prominent anxiety symptoms

52 Common psychiatric disorders as seen in primary care:
(a) Occur in 50% of women within a year
(b) Seldom respond to counselling
(c) Should always be referred to a psychiatrist
(d) Often present with physical symptoms
(e) Usually have a florid presentation

53 Community care of patients with severe psychiatric illness:
(a) Is cheaper than institutional care
(b) Requires detailed care planning
(c) Is formalized in the 1987 Care in the Community Act
(d) Has to be based in community mental health centres
(e) Can prevent institutionalization

54 Fitness to plead requires:
(a) Literacy
(b) Understanding of the nature of the charges being faced
(c) Capacity to instruct counsel
(d) The absence of current psychotic features
(e) Understanding of the meaning of a guilty plea

55 Predictors of violence in offenders include:
(a) Past violence
(b) Masochistic fantasies
(c) Impulsivity
(d) Cyclothymic personality
(e) Learning disability

56 The following statements concerning the 1983 Mental Health Act (England and Wales) are true:
(a) Section 2 lasts for up to 6 months
(b) Section 41 restricted patients may not be discharged without the Prime Minister's consent
(c) Consent to ECT is covered in Section 58
(d) Patients on Section 3 can only go on leave with the written consent of the Responsible Medical Officer
(e) Mental illness is not defined within the Act

57 Compulsory admission under the 1983 Mental Health Act (England and Wales) requires:
(a) Current mental illness
(b) Dangerousness
(c) Refusal of voluntary admission or treatment
(d) The presence of the patient's GP
(e) Application by a social worker

58 Common sexual dysfunctions in men include:
(a) Lack of sexual enjoyment
(b) Ejaculatory failure
(c) Pain on intercourse
(d) Fetishism
(e) Transsexuality

59 Variations of the sexual act include:
(a) Exhibitionism
(b) Paedophilia
(c) Frotteurism
(d) Necrophilia
(e) Dyspareunia

60 The following statements about HIV are true:
(a) The worldwide death toll is approximately 5 million
(b) Acute stress reactions are common
(c) Self-help groups can play an important role
(d) AZT can induce schizophrenia
(e) Parietal hypoperfusion is characteristic of HIV-I associated dementia

61 Psychoanalysis:
(a) Stresses the importance of childhood experience
(b) Is indicated in bipolar disorders
(c) Requires the ability to cope with painful insights
(d) Was introduced by Carl Jung
(e) Relies on the countertransference

62 Interpersonal psychotherapy (IPT):
(a) Was devised by Sigmund Freud
(b) Is indicated for psychotic depression
(c) Has role transition as a focus
(d) Is useful in eating disorders
(e) Links interpersonal difficulties with severity of depression

63 Phenothiazines:
   (a) Block cholinergic receptors
   (b) Cause menorrhagia
   (c) Are excreted intact in the urine
   (d) Seldom cause tardive dyskinesia
   (e) Are associated with haemolytic jaundice

64 Selective serotonin reuptake inhibitors:
   (a) Are only indicated in the treatment of depressive disorders
   (b) Are usually given by injection
   (c) Achieve a response rate of 90% in clinical practice
   (d) Often cause headache
   (e) Often cause dry mouth

65 Indications for ECT include:
   (a) Cotard's syndrome
   (b) Catatonia
   (c) Anxiety
   (d) Puerperal psychosis
   (e) Fregoli's syndrome

66 Side effects of lithium include:
   (a) Oedema
   (b) Hyperthyroidism
   (c) Diarrhoea
   (d) Fine tremor
   (e) Leucopenia

67 Benzodiazepines:
   (a) Should not be given to people with epilepsy
   (b) May induce tolerance
   (c) Inhibit the excitatory effects of GABA
   (d) Are indicated in the treatment of alcohol withdrawal
   (e) Potentiate alcohol

68 The following statements about cross-cultural syndromes are true:
   (a) Amok is a response to humiliation
   (b) Echopraxia is a central feature of Koro
   (c) Dissociative features are frequently found
   (d) Latah is frequently found in South America
   (e) Hyperventilation may precipitate 'Ataque de nervios'

69 Tourette's syndrome:
   (a) Is characterized by multiple tics
   (b) Responds well to benzodiazepines
   (c) More often affects men than women
   (d) Is associated with early maternal separation
   (e) Usually presents in early adult life

70 The following statements about unusual psychiatric syndromes are true:
   (a) de Clerambault's syndrome may be a feature of mania
   (b) The main risk in Othello syndrome is of suicide
   (c) Delusional parasitosis was first described by Ganser
   (d) Couvade syndrome is a form of delusional misidentification
   (e) In *Folie a deux*, both victims have a psychotic illness